Introduction to Resear[ch] Data Analysis in the He[alth]

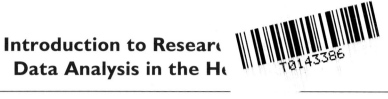

The 'health sciences' are a broad and diverse area. Health sciences include public health, primary care, health psychology, psychiatry and epidemiology. The research methods and data analysis skills required across them, however, are very similar. Moreover, the ability to *appraise* and *conduct* research is emphasised within the health sciences – and students are expected increasingly to do both.

Introduction to Research Methods and Data Analysis in the Health Sciences presents a balanced blend of quantitative research methods, and the most widely used techniques for collecting and analysing data in the health sciences. Highly practical in nature, the book guides you, step by step, through the research process, and covers both the consumption and the production of research and data analysis. Divided into the three strands that run throughout quantitative health science research – critical numbers, critical appraisal of existing research, and conducting new research – this accessible textbook introduces:

- Descriptive statistics
- Measures of association for categorical and continuous outcomes
- Confounding, effect modification, mediation and causal inference
- Critical appraisal
- Searching the literature
- Randomised controlled trials
- Cohort studies
- Case-control studies
- Research ethics and data management
- Dissemination and publication
- Linear regression for continuous outcomes
- Logistic regression for categorical outcomes.

A dedicated companion website offers additional teaching and learning resources for students and lecturers, including screenshots, R programming code, and extensive self-assessment material linked to the book's exercises and activities.

Clear and accessible with a comprehensive coverage to equip the reader with an understanding of the research process and the practical skills they need to collect and analyse data, it is essential reading for all undergraduate and postgraduate students in the health and medical sciences.

Gareth Hagger-Johnson is a Senior Research Associate in the Department of Epidemiology and Public Health at University College London, UK.

Introduction to Research Methods and Data Analysis in the Health Sciences

Gareth Hagger-Johnson

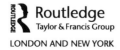

Routledge
Taylor & Francis Group

LONDON AND NEW YORK

First published 2014
by Routledge
2 Park Square, Milton Park, Abingdon, Oxon, OX14 4RN

and by Routledge
711 Third Avenue, New York, NY 10017

Routledge is an imprint of the Taylor & Francis Group, an informa business

British Library Cataloguing in Publication Data
A catalogue record for this book is available from the British Library

Library of Congress Cataloging-in-Publication Data
Hagger-Johnson, Gareth, author.
Introduction to research methods and data analysis in the health
sciences / Gareth Hagger-Johnson.
    p. ; cm.
 I. Title.
 [DNLM: 1. Biomedical Research--methods. 2. Data Interpretation,
 Statistical. 3. Research Design. W 20.5]
 R850
 610.72'4--dc23   2013048268

ISBN13: 978-0-415-73408-0 (hbk)
ISBN13: 978-0-273-76384-0 (pbk)
ISBN13: 978-1-315-77111-3 (ebk)

Typeset in Palatino by
HWA Text and Data Management, London

For Ari

Contents

Contents

Figures

Tables

Boxes

Contents

Acknowledgements

I would like to thank Laura Stroud, Graham Law and the many students at University of Leeds who provided feedback on earlier versions of learning exercises in this book. As always, my friends and family have been an enormous source of support. Finally, I would like to thank colleagues and students at UCL Department of Epidemiology and Public Health and UCL Institute of Child Health.

Part I

Introduction

Evidence-based health research

The term 'health sciences' is broad, referring to public health, primary care, health psychology, psychiatry and epidemiology. Students in the health sciences are not necessarily aligned to any one discipline. However, there are large numbers of students taking health sciences courses. Although the courses taken tend to differ, the research methods and data analysis skills required are very similar. In most cases, courses require students to:

1 locate, understand existing research

2 appraise existing research

3 design, collect and analyse data from their own research.

There are four themes in health sciences learning and teaching which have all become more prominent in recent years [5]:

- evidence-based practice

- research-based learning

- learning research methods

- linking staff research activity and teaching.

Evidence-based practice is perhaps the most prominent change within the health sciences in recent years. It is defined as the 'process of systematically finding, appraising and using contemporaneous research findings as the basis for clinical decisions' [6]. Originating from 'evidence-based medicine' [7], it is characterised by a shift from relying on internal knowledge, to relying on both internal and external knowledge:

Internal evidence is composed of knowledge acquired through formal education and training, general experience accumulated from daily practice, and specific experience gained from an individual clinician-patient relationship. External evidence is accessible information from research. It is the explicit use of valid external evidence (eg, randomised controlled trials) combined with the prevailing internal evidence that defines a clinical decision as 'evidence-based'. [8]

The evidence-based approach is becoming the norm in the health sciences [5], as is the requirement for students to produce their own evidence. Very few books are available which cover both the consumption and the production of research (see Table 1.1 below). More typically, books will either address epidemiology, statistics and critical appraisal (consumption) or research design and data analysis (production) – rarely both.

Currently, students in the health sciences tend to rely on *ad hoc* combinations of textbooks from nursing, medicine, psychology and social sciences. Existing books rarely offer the breadth and depth to cover health sciences in its entirety, while still appealing to specific subject areas. Health sciences are multidisciplinary, which presents challenges for any book trying to introduce students to research methods covering such diverse areas. However, this book aims to capture the three important strands than run through health sciences research: statistics, critical appraisal and conducting new research. Again, the ability to appraise and conduct research is becoming more strongly emphasised in the health sciences – students need to learn how to do both, but are rarely offered a single book that shows them how.

The book is aimed at postgraduate students studying courses in the health sciences, chiefly in the UK (since many readers will work for the NHS) but also internationally. It should also be relevant for:

- medical undergraduates (e.g. epidemiology, critical appraisal, statistics)
- research students
  - ordinary PhD students
  - doctoral students in clinical psychology

Health sciences students have very different backgrounds, and few assumptions can be made about their level of existing knowledge. Unlike vocational subjects, health sciences are drawn from very different levels of experience. This book tries not to make too many assumptions.

In my experience, students in the health sciences have two key concerns – their summative assessment and their requirement to analyse data using appropriate statistical software. The book will support students by linking the exercises and activities to formative assessment (in MCQ format) on the book website. Given that student learning is driven by assessment, I hope that students will appreciate having available a formative tool to guide their learning. Formative assessment allows students to take control of their own learning [9], in preparation for summative assessment.

The second concern is particularly relevant for health sciences students. Many health sciences students work in the NHS or voluntary/community sector, and do not have access to popular statistical packages such as Stata or SPSS (these require a licence). To address the second issue, this book makes reference to the open source statistical package called R. Although this is less familiar to many readers, it is growing in popularity, as evidenced by the number of books now available on R. As an open source package, it requires no licence fee and can be run on any PC or Mac. The book and supporting website contain screenshots and R programming code. I do not think that students should have to spend any additional money simply in order to run their statistical models.

Preliminary exercise and installing R

This preliminary chapter includes a simple formative numeracy exercise, which you can use to decide whether you need to refresh your memory of basic mathematics. It also contains instructions for downloading and installing R, a program which will be used throughout the book as a calculator, for statistical analysis, and for making graphs.

Intended learning outcomes

By the end of this chapter, you should be able to:

- complete a formative numeracy exercise
- identify areas of numerical skill that you need to improve
- download and install the R software
- perform basic calculations using the R software.

Before reading on, you may find it useful to complete a quick formative numeracy exercise. This will help you identify numeracy skills that you need to learn or revisit. The exercise is adapted from a standard measure of numeracy scale, used in research settings [10]. Don't worry if you can't answer them all. Several of the questions involve concepts that will be introduced in the next few chapters, and there will be plenty of opportunity to practise them.

Box 1.1 Exercise: Formative numeracy exercise (adapted from [11]).

1 Imagine that we have a fair, six-sided die (for example, from a board game or a casino craps table). Imagine we now roll it 1000 times. Out of 1000 rolls, how many times do you think the die would come up even (numbers 2, 4, or 6)?

2 In the Big Bucks Lottery, the chance of winning a $10.00 prize is 1%. What is your best guess about how many people would win a $10.00 prize if 1000 people each buy a single ticket to Big Bucks?

---

3   In the Acme Publishing Sweepstakes, the chance of winning a car is 1 in 1000. What percentage of tickets to Acme Publishing Sweepstakes win a car?

4   Which of the following numbers represents the biggest risk of getting a disease?

   a   1 in 100

   b   1 in 1000

   c   1 in 10

5   Which of the following numbers represents the biggest risk of getting a disease?

   a   1%

   b   10%

   c   5%

6   If person A's risk of getting a disease is 1% in 10 years, and person B's risk is double that of A's, what is B's risk?

7   If person A's chance of getting a disease is 1 in 100 in 10 years, and person B's risk is double that of A's, what is B's risk?

8   If the chance of getting a disease is 10%, how many people out of 100 would be expected to get the disease?

9   If the chance of getting a disease is 10%, how many people out of 1000 would be expected to get the disease?

10 The chance of getting a viral infection is 0.0005. Out of 10,000 people, about how many of them are expected to get infected?

Answers can be found towards the end of this chapter.

How to install the R program

The R program is the software used throughout this book. R is an open source program, meaning that it has no licence fee. R can be used both as a calculator (for example, in this chapter) and for statistical analysis (in later chapters). R is increasingly popular in many health sciences, particularly epidemiology and biostatistics. It is a good idea to install R at this stage, and practise some basic calculations, in order to become familiar and comfortable with the R interface.

Installing R

You can install R on your own PC or laptop relatively easily. If you are working at the university, hospital or other organisation, check with your IT support team. Not all organisations allow software to be downloaded without restriction, as a security precaution.

1 Visit the R website at http://cran.r-project.org

2 Click on Download R for your platform (e.g. Windows, Mac or Linux).

The Comprehensive R Archive Network

CRAN
Mirrors
What's new?
Task Views
Search

About R
R Homepage
The R

Download and Install R

Precompiled binary distributions of the base system and contributed packages, **Windows and Mac** users most likely want one of these versions of R:

- Download R for Linux
- Download R for (Mac) OS X
- Download R for Windows

Figure 1.1 Comprehensive R Archive Network download page

3 Now click on base or click install R for the first time.

4 The most recent version of the software will be displayed. R is updated regularly. Click on the Download R link, which will also show the version number and the platform you chose at step 2.

5 Double click on the file you have downloaded (ending in .exe) to start the installation.

6 You will be asked to choose a language (e.g. English), click Next to continue, read the GNU general public license information (click Next to continue) and then choose a location to install the software. For readers using a PC, typically, the location is C:\Program Files\R\ followed by the most recent version number, but other locations can be chosen.

7 You will then be asked to choose which component you want to install. The default setting (32-bit user installation) is fine for most purposes including all of the examples used in this book.

8 On the next screen, you can choose to customise the start-up options, but you can select No here to accept the default settings. You are also asked where R should place the program's shortcuts. For readers using a PC, the default suggestion (a folder called R in the Start Menu folder) is fine, so click Next to continue.

9   Finally, you can choose whether to have R shortcuts on the desktop (click Next).

10 When the installation has been completed successfully, you will see a message confirming that R has finished installing. Click Finish to complete the process.

Starting R

When you have installed R, for readers using a PC, it can be opened using the start menu or double clicking the program icon in the Program Files folder or location that you chosen during the installation.

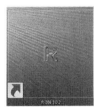

Figure 1.2 R program icon

1   When you open R, the interface shown is called the R graphical user interface (GUI, pronounced 'gooey'). This is simply called the 'interface' hereafter.

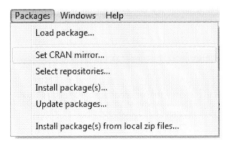

Figure 1.3 Selecting CRAN mirror

2   The first thing to do each time you open R is choose a local Comprehensive R Archive Network (CRAN) 'mirror' that will allow you to download and install the different 'packages' that you will use. Choose the location nearest to you (e.g. London, Bristol). We might assume that locations nearby will download packages faster, although faster download speeds in recent years have made this kind of choice less important.

3   The second thing to do each time you open R is to set the local working directory. This is very important, because R needs to know where your

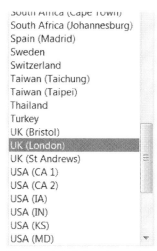

Figure 1.4 Selecting mirror location

data files will be located. You may prefer to use the desktop, or My Documents, a USB storage device, or some other location. As an example, to set the desktop as the working directory, click on File, Change dir… and then locate the desktop. You may have to type the location manually (e.g. C:\Users\Gareth\Desktop) and click on OK. The interface is now ready for use.

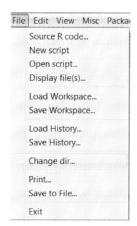

Figure 1.5 Setting working directory

Box 1.2 Exercise: Simple equation.
Note down your answer to the following equation:

    $4 + 5 \times 8 = ?$

Did you get 44 or 72? You might well have reached either answer, depending on how your approached the equation. If you did 5×8 first, then added 4, this would give 44. If you did $4 + 5$ first and then multiplied by 8, this would have given 72. The fact that two answers can be reached illustrates the need to have some rule, or order of operations. The BODMAS rule is provided for exactly this reason. It stands for brackets, orders, division, multiplication, addition and subtraction. The list is the order in which you should approach an equation, working from left to right. If you follow this order, you will arrive at the correct answer. In our example, the correct answer was 44. We should have done the multiplication first (5×8) and then addition (add 4), according to the BODMAS rule. This gives the answer of 44. To avoid an ambiguity, researchers will sometimes add brackets for you, but not always.

    A second convention which can help avoid ambiguity is to avoid using the times ($\times$) symbol altogether. This may seem strange to those of you who are used to using the mathematical symbols $\times$, $\div$, + and $-$. The problem is, the symbol x is usually reserved for referring to a variable (as in x, y or z). The x usually represents a variable, and should not be confused with a multiplication sign. Multiplication and division do not need symbols, because the need to multiply or divide should be clear from the context. For example when working by hand using an equation, xy means multiply x and y together. x/z means divide x by z. There is no need to have a separate symbol for multiply or divide. In Excel and in R, the symbols used are + (addition), $-$ (subtraction), * (multiplication) and / (division).

Basic calculations in R

R can be used for basic calculations. For example, to work out the answer to $4 + 5 \times 8$, you can type 4+5*8 as shown in the Figure 1.6. This gives the correct answer of 44. If you wanted to specify that 4+5 should be performed first, you can simply add brackets to make this clear. A useful list of arithmetic operators is shown in Table 1.1.

```
> 4+5*8
[1] 44
> (4+5)*8
[1] 72
> |
```

Figure 1.6 Performing a calculation in R

Table 1.1 List of arithmetical operators

Arithmetic operator	Description	Example	Result
+	Add	4+5	9
−	Subtract	2–5	–3
*	Multiply	8*6	48
/	Divide	1/2	0.5
^	Exponentiate (raise to a power)	4^2	16

Throughout the book, R code is shown in a box, with a `monospaced font` for the specific code that should be entered into the program. It is assumed that you will then 'Enter' to run any piece of code. Comments are often provided at the end of the code, after hash symbol #. R will ignore anything that is after a hash symbol, so it does not matter if you include these comments or not. Their purpose is simply to help you understand what each line of code is doing.

> **Box 1.3** An aside: numbers raised to a power
> It is important to familiarise yourself with numbers raised to a power, if you are not already familiar. The following apology appeared in *The Independent* newspaper (13 September 2008), following an error that appeared in a report about the launch of the Hadron Collider:
> 'Last week, a formatting error led to us inadvertently suggesting that there was a one in 1,019 chance of the world ending before this edition. That should have read, er, one in 10^{19} – rather less likely. Sorry. Feel free to remove the crash helmet'.

Answers to the formative numeracy exercise using R

The answers to the formative numeracy exercise above are now explained, together with examples of R code for doing these calculations.

1 Three out of six sides of a dice are even numbers, so you could think of this as a fraction and convert it into a decimal, multiplying by 1000. `3/6*1000 # or equivalently 1/2*1000, since 3/6 is the same as 1/2`.

2 One out of every 100 people win, and 1000 buy a ticket, so `1/100*1000`. = 10.

3 One in 1000 as a decimal is 1/1000, which as a percentage is `.0001*100`. = 0.1%.

4 This is fairly straightforward without needing to do any calculations, but if you wanted to convert all three fractions to decimals this might help you to visualise which is the largest.

```
a 1/100 # 1/100 = 0.1
b 1/1000 # 1/1000 = 0.001
c 1/10 # 1/10 = 0.1, which is clearly the largest.
```

5 This should not require any calculations, because it is clear that 10% is the largest risk.

6 To double the risk, simply multiply the figure by 2. 1% if 1/100 so `1/100*2` = 0.02 or 2%.

7 This is the same as question 6. Both refer to the same time period (10 years) but the risk is exactly the same in both scenarios (1%).

8 This is fairly straightforward. `10/100*100` = 10.

9 This happens to be the same percentage as question 7, but is a different calculation. `10/100*1000`.= 100.

10 This question involves multiplying the probability of the event by the number of people at risk (`0.0005*10000` = 5).

Summary of answers: (1) 500; (2) 10; (3) 0.1%; (4) c; (5) b; (6) 2% in 10 years; (7) 2 in 10 in 10 years; (8) 10; (9) 100; (10) 0.0005*10000 = 5. Question 10 is the most difficult question. It involves thinking about probability, multiplication and proportions. In Chapter 2, we will introduce proportions and rates in more detail.

You can use this exercise to identify which numeracy skills require revision. For example, many students find question 10 the most difficult, since it involves decimals, probability, multiplication and is not intuitive. You may find the Table 1.2 useful for refreshing your memory about decimals, fractions and percentages.

Further reading

Evidence-based health research:

Long A, Harrison S, Evidence-Based Decision Making. *Health Service Journal* 1997, S6:1–11.

Basic mathematics and numeracy:

Bittinger M, *Basic College Mathematics*. London: Pearson Education, 2009.
Johnson T, Neill H, *Teach Yourself Mathematics*, 3rd edn. London: Teach Yourself, 2008.

R

Allerhand M, *A Tiny Handbook of R* (SpringerBriefs in Statistics). Heidelberg: Springer, 2011.
Crawley M, *The R Book*. Chichester: Wiley, 2012.
Field A, Miles J, Field Z, *Discovering Statistics Using R*. Thousand Oaks, CA: SAGE Publications Ltd, 2012.

Table 1.2 Decimals, fractions and percentages

Decimal	Fraction	Percentage
0.01	1/100	1%
0.05	1/20	5%
0.1	1/10	10%
0.2	1/5	20%
0.25	1/4	25%
0.333333...	1/3	33.33...%
0.5	1/2	50%
0.75	3/4	75%
0.9	9/10	90%
1.0	NA	100%
1.1	11/10	110%
1.25	5/4	125%

Table 1.3 Relational operators in R

Relational operators in R	Description
==	Equal to
<	Less than
<=	Less than or equal to
>	Greater than
>=	Greater than or equal to
!=	Not equal to

Part II

Critical numbers

Descriptive statistics part I

Levels of measurement and measures of central tendency

Descriptive statistics are an important preliminary step prior to any statistical analysis. They are also important in their own right for people who want to make sense of the results. Well-presented descriptive statistics (or simply 'descriptives', a popular shorthand) communicate important features of the data. They tell the reader which variables were included in the study, their units of measurement, their range, and their frequency or distribution. Descriptives are the first thing to concentrate on when conducting your own research, and when appraising others' research, which we will do in later chapters.

Intended learning outcomes

By the end of this chapter, you should be able to:

- identify the level of measurement for a variable
- define and calculate proportions
- define and calculate measures of central tendency
    - mean
    - median
    - mode
    - range

Introducing key terms

It is important to define key terms that will be used throughout this book. Suppose that the table below represents some data we have collected as part of a research study. The table represents a data set, and this might be stored in a data file (for example, an MS Excel spreadsheet or a comma separated file for R). The cells in the data set contain the data values, and these are the realised measurements. Put simply, the cells contain our data. The columns represent

Table 2.1 Sample data

ID	Sex	Height (cm)
1	2	168.7
2	1	172.0
3	1	176.5
4	1	160.5
5	2	174.0
6	1	168.6
7	2	160.0
8	2	163.0
9	1	175.0
10	2	161.4

variables, the characteristics being measured. The rows represent participants in the study, also known as cases or observations. These are the people who we have observed in our study. Finally, measurement is the process by which we got our data. We might have used a ruler to measure height, and a questionnaire for people to self-report their sex. The ID number would have been assigned sequentially, starting with the first participant who joined the study.

Levels of measurement

Different variables produce data with different levels of measurement. Broadly speaking, there are two types of data: categorical or continuous. There are different types of categorical and continuous data, which we will explore in more detail below. Categorical data are usually described by presenting the number of people in a category, and the percentage of people this represented. Continuous data are usually described using some measure of central tendency and some measure of dispersion (both are terms described properly below). When doing your own research, deciding whether data are categorical or continuous is very important, because it determines the type of statistics which are appropriate to use. This is particularly important for 'outcome' variables in a study, that is, variables which we think should change following an intervention, or which are changed by some exposure (see Chapter 4).

Categorical data

Four types of data are ranked from the lowest level of measurement, to the highest: nominal, ordinal, interval and ratio.

Nominal data

Nominal data can be classified into mutually exclusive categories. That is, each person can belong to one category only. Examples include vital status (dead, alive), ethnic minority status (minority, not a minority), method of travelling to work (bus, car, train, walk, other) incidence of coronary heart disease (yes, no). Sex is usually recorded as male or female, but there have been calls to allow transgender persons to report their gender differently. Nominal data that have only two categories are called binary data. Example includes yes/no, present/absent, and pass/fail.

Ordinal data

Ordinal data are similar to nominal data in that each person can only belong to one category. The categories, however, are ranked in a meaningful way. For example, in a marathon race, athletes might come first, second, or third. This way of recording the measurements produces ordinal data. We know the order in which runners finished the race, but nothing more. We did not record finishing time, or any more detail than their race position. Ordinal data provides more information than nominal data, because it is possible to make comparisons. For example, I could say that the runner finishing second was slower than the one finishing first, but faster than the one finishing third.

Continuous data

Continuous data are measured on a scale, with meaningful distance information between the points. There are two types of continuous data: interval and ratio.

Interval data

Interval data (sometimes called discrete data) contains meaningful distance information. The intervals between points are equidistant, and the values are not restricted in the way that ordinal data are. It is possible to perform addition and subtraction on an interval scale. It is also possible to have negative values, unlike with ordinal data. It is important to note however, that there is no true zero point on an interval scale. This means that multiplication and division are not possible on an interval scale. Examples include degrees Celsius and degrees Fahrenheit. Both are interval scales, but neither has a true zero point. It is incorrect to claim that 40 degrees Celsius is twice as hot as 20 degrees Celsius, because this calculation implies some zero point.

Likert scales, which ask respondents to a questionnaire to endorse response options such as 'strongly agree' to 'strongly disagree' are often thought of as interval level. This is controversial,

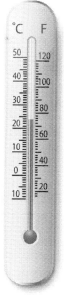

Figure 2.1 Interval data

and may depend on the number of response options, among other issues. Psychologists have suggested that Likert scales should have at least five and preferably seven options, in order to be reasonably treated as interval data. The more response options, the more normally distributed (a term introduced below) the data are likely to be.

Ratio data

It is not until we reach the ratio level of measurement that multiplication and division are possible. Ratio data have a true zero point. For example, degrees Kelvin are recorded on a truly ratio scale, where zero really does represent the absence of temperature. Out of interest, 0 degrees Kelvin is equivalent to –273.15 Celsius. You might wonder why we bother having 0 degrees Celsius at all, if Kelvin has useful measurement properties and a true zero point. This is clearly for convenience, because 0 degrees Celsius (273.15 Kelvin) happens to be the point at which water freezes. It does not imply that there is no temperature at 0 degrees Celsius. Other examples of ratio level data are speed, time, weight, height, probability (risk) and odds. These latter two terms are introduced in the next chapter. Multiplication and division are perfectly permissible with these kinds of data, because all have a true zero point. There are other useful things we can do with continuous data, particularly statistical techniques. Several statistical techniques assume that your data are ratio level, which is one reason why it is so important to clarify exactly what level of measurement your data have.

Although I have described levels of measurement as ranging from lowest (nominal) to highest (ratio), this should not imply that they range from worst to best. The level of measurement depends entirely on what is appropriate for the variable concerned, and the research question. There are also situations in which you may decide to change your level of measurement. Indeed, several examples appear in this book, such as the decision to categorise body mass index (BMI) into specific categories (underweight, normal weight, overweight, obese). This is useful in many different situations, but you must be clear about what the level of measurement was to begin with, and what you have changed it to. Generally speaking, there are a greater range of statistical techniques available for continuous data than for categorical data. In Chapter 13, the importance of collecting data as continuous is emphasised, so that data are preserved with as much detail as possible. There are several different reasons why this is useful, but none imply that ratio data are necessarily 'better' than categorical data. I should also point out that the four different levels of measurement are not as unambiguous as I have implied here. This is illustrated in Exercise 2.1.

Box 2.1 Exercise: Levels of measurement 1

See if you can identify the level of measurement for each of the following variables. Tick one box only for each variable, then check your answers on the book website. Note that not all of these variables can be clearly identified as belonging to one level of measurement only – it sometimes depends on the context. Indeed, the purpose of this exercise is to sensitise you to the ambiguity that can arise when attempting to decide if your data are categorical or continuous. There is not always a clear answer.

Variable	Categorical		Continuous	
Level of measurement	Nominal	Ordinal	Interval	Ratio
Stage of cancer classified as stage I to IV				
Age (years)				
Serum cholesterol (mg/dL)				
HIV status (positive or negative)				
Score on the Glasgow Coma Scale (which ranges from 3 to 15)				
Smoker (current, former, non-smoker)				
CHD onset (yes or no)				
BMI (weight in kgs/height in metres^2)				
Weight (kg)				
Temperature (Celsius)				
Temperature (Kelvin)				
ID number given to volunteers in a study				
General Health Questionnaire score (a measure of anxiety and depression)				
Patient reported outcome measure (PROM) on a Likert scale (strongly agree = 5, strongly disagree = 1)				

Table 2.2 Permissible statements for each level of measurement

Level	Permissible statements	Statistics
Nominal	=, ≠	Mode
Ordinal	=, ≠, <, >	Median
Interval	=, ≠, <, >, +, −	(Arithmetic) mean, standard deviation
Ratio	=, ≠, <, >, +, −, ×, ÷	Geometric mean, coefficient of variation

Why is determining the level of measurement important?

The statistical analysis that can be performed on data depends on the level of measurement. It is important to clarify what the level of measurement actually is, because this will determine what statistics are appropriate. In the next chapter, basic descriptive statistics are introduced which are only suitable if we know what the level of measurement is. In Table 2.2 is a summary of the permissible statements for these kinds of data for each level of measurement

The geometric mean and coefficients of variation are not covered in this book, but are included in the table for completeness. In most cases, when people use the term 'mean' they actually refer to the arithmetic mean. For the remainder of this book, the same convention is adopted. The key point to remember is that the higher the level of measurement, the more operations can be performed. The statistics which can be used are shown in the rightmost column and are introduced below.

Box 2.2 Exercise: Levels of measurement 2

See if you can identify the levels of measurement in this extract. The variables are highlighted in bold for you. Check your answers on the book website.

The dwarfing apple rootstock '**M27**' was raised in **1929** from a cross between '**M9**' and '**M13**'. As a dwarf bush, it makes a tree **1.2 to 1.5m** in height and spread. A well-grown apple tree should yield on average **4.5 to 6.8kg** of fruit each year. At planting, side-shoots are cut back to **three buds** and the leader pruned by about **one quarter**, cutting to an upward facing bud.

([17], p. 56)

Are levels of measurement potentially misleading?

Some commentators have argued that dividing data into 'types' (nominal, ordinal, discrete, continuous) can be misleading. It is not always possible to choose the appropriate level of measurement. For example, suppose that in a raffle ticket number 24 has won a prize. These are four responses from different people who have entered the raffle:

- Grace: 'I can only win or lose, and have lost.'
- Ruby: 'It doesn't look like there are 24 people here.'
- Olivia: 'I arrived too soon.'
- Emily: 'If I knew the rate and regularity of arrivals, I could have arrived at the right time.'

You can probably tell that each person has a different level of measurement in mind, when they think about their ticket in relation to the winning ticket. Grace has adopted nominal level thinking (win or lose). Ruby looks around and says 'It doesn't look like there are 24 people here', interpreting the number as interval level. Olivia compares her number (23) to winning number (24) and says 'I arrived too soon'. This shows ordinal level thinking. Emily wondered if she could work out the rate and regularity of arrivals, she could have arrived at the right time. This is ratio level thinking, because Emily is thinking of the variable time, rather than the order in which people arrived. This example illustrates that nominal, ordinal, interval and ratio typologies can sometimes mislead [18]. In reality, the distinction between levels of measurement is not clear-cut and is a choice made by the researcher, or conventions adopted by a particular research community.

## 3

Descriptive statistics part 2

Measures of dispersion

Intended learning outcomes

By the end of this chapter, you should be able to define and calculate measures of dispersion:

- variance
- standard deviation
- standard error.

The purpose of statistics is to simplify the presentation of data, often complex data, in a way that makes them easier to understand. Although they may seem complicated to the beginner, statistics does make appraising and conducting research easier, not more difficult. Statistical modelling is a useful term, invoking that researchers are making models of their data, as simplified representations of the real thing. Some models are more complicated than others. And some models are more accurate than others. In a statistical model, there is a balance to be made between presenting a simple model and presenting an accurate model. If it is too simple, it may be wrong. If it is too accurate, it may be too complicated to understand and communicate. In the example in Table 3.1, a small data set is shown. As with all data sets in this book, it is available for download on the book website. There are ten participants in the study, and their height was recorded in centimetres. On the right hand side is a model of the data. This is not a very good statistical model, because it has not been simplified. Put differently, it is not parsimonious. There are ten data points in the original data set and ten in the model. The model is equally complex as the original data [19]. Although it is an accurate model, data sets are frequently very large and making copies of them is not practical. Researchers might consider presenting results from a small case study in this way, but what if the study contained 10,000 participants? Clearly, a simpler model of the data is required.

Table 3.1 Example data set

ID	Height (cm)	Model
1	168.70	168.70
2	172.00	172.00
3	176.50	176.50
4	160.50	160.50
5	174.00	174.00
6	168.60	168.60
7	160.00	160.00
8	163.00	163.00
9	175.00	175.00
10	161.40	161.40

Mean

The model we present to the audience is a choice, and it is important to make the right choice, because some models are better than others. A good statistical model is first and foremost simpler than the original data. It should also make the most of the data, making full use of what is available. Clearly, it would be a waste of time and resources to collect data that is not actually used. Finally, a model should communicate the right story, and not a misleading story that hides or amplifies particular features. So can we make a model of our data that has less than ten pieces of information? We can model the central tendency of the data by calculating the mean or the average height. We can calculate the average height, simply by adding (or summing) the data values and dividing by the sample size which is ten:

$$(168.7 + 172 + 176.5 + 160.5 + 174 + 168.6 + 160 + 163 + 175 + 161.4)/10 = 168.0$$

This is called the mean height. The mean height is 168.0 cm, which is a good model of these data. Strictly speaking, this statistic is called the arithmetic mean because there are other types of means available, which aren't discussed

---

Box 3.1 R code to calculate the mean

After loading in the heights data, you can request the mean using the simple function mean(x) where x is the name of the variable.

```
data <- read.table('height.csv', header=TRUE, sep=',')
#Note that the <- symbol is used to tell R that the data is
#in the table.
attach(data)
mean(height)
```

---

here. The mean, then, is a model that simplifies the data. It is a descriptive statistic which in this example, can summarise ten pieces of information using only one number.

Sample and population mean

The sample mean is an estimate of the mean in the population from which the sample was taken.

Larger sample sizes will provide a mean that is closer to the population mean (μ). Very small samples are more likely to under- or over-estimate the true population mean. As the sample size becomes very large, there is no benefit to having larger sample sizes. The sample mean becomes almost exactly the same as the population mean. Clearly, if a sample was so large that it included the entire population, the sample mean and the population mean would be exactly the same. There are methods for determining the appropriate sample size, discussed in Chapter 11.

Median

The median is also a model of the central tendency in a set of data. The median is the middle value, but only if the data have been sorted, as they have been here. It is the value that divides a distribution in half. If someone has been kind enough to sort your data for you (Table 3.2), you can find the median by taking the middle observation (if the data have an odd number), or the average of two middle ones (if the data have an even number, as they do here). The median is also the 50th percentile, if the data are divided into 100 percentage points. In this example, the median height is (after rounding up), 168.7. So is the median a good model here? It is certainly simpler than the data, because it is one value

Table 3.2 Calculating the median

ID sorted from smallest to largest	Height (cm)
7	160.0
4	160.5
10	161.4
8	163.0
6	168.6
1	168.7
2	172.0
5	174.0
9	175.0
3	176.5
Median	168.7

Table 3.3 Comparing the mean and the median

ID	Annual salary (£)
1	12,000
2	13,000
3	12,000
4	100,000
5	15,000
6	13,000
7	12,500
8	9,000
9	13,500
10	24,000

and the data has 10 values. However, it only uses one or perhaps two of the data points, out of all of the data that has been collected. The mean is often preferred to the median for this reason; because the mean takes into account all of the data values. And yet, in our example, the median tells the same story as the mean – that the average person is about 168cm tall. This is not the case for all data – the median can often tell a very different story to the mean.

Box 3.2 An aside: misleading medians

Stephen Jay Gould wrote that he was diagnosed with cancer in 1982. The doctor told him that the cancer was incurable, with a median mortality of eight months after discovery:

> When I learned about the eight-month median, my first intellectual reaction was: fine, half the people will live longer; now what are my chances of being in that half. I read for a furious and nervous hour and concluded, with relief: damned good. I possessed every one of the characteristics conferring a probability of longer life: I was young; my disease had been recognised in a relatively early stage; I would receive the nation's best medical treatment; I had the world to live for; I knew how to read the data properly and not despair. Another technical point then added even more solace. I immediately recognised that the distribution of variation about the eight-month median would almost surely be what statisticians call 'right skewed.' (http://www.stat.berkeley.edu/users/rice/Stat2/GouldCancer.html)

In fact, Gould died 20 years later, so he was correct not to adopt the median (eight months) as the best model for his own survival time.

The example in Table 3.3 helps to illustrate important differences between the mean and the median. Suppose you saw a recruitment poster, which claimed that the average salary was £22,400. This is correct, because the mean salary is £22,400. But is it a good model of the data? Again, it is simpler than the data, and it uses all of the available data, but it tells a misleading story. The relatively high salary of £100,000 has skewed the distribution of income values, pulling the mean away from the centre of the distribution. The median is still the middle value, which is a better measure of the central tendency in this example. The median salary is just £13,000.

Mode

The mode is another measure of central tendency. The mode is the most frequently occurring value. In the example in Table 3.4, the modal hospital stay is two days. It is rare to see the mode reported in the literature. Although it is simpler than the data, in our example it only makes use of four values. And in many data sets, there is no mode. It does tell the right story here, because most people stay for two days, or something else. The median is three, which doesn't really reflect the typical or most frequent length of stay.

Table 3.4 Calculating the mode

ID	Length of hospital stay (days)
1	2
2	2
3	2
4	1
5	3
6	3
7	28
8	7
9	21
10	2

Range

The range is sometimes used to summarise data. To calculate the range, sort the data, and note the smallest (minimum) value and the largest (maximum) value. Subtracting the minimum from the maximum (in other words, the difference between them) gives the range. In the example in Table 3.5, the range is £91,000. Is the range a good model? It is simpler than the data, uses two values, and could tell a misleading story. It does not give a clear indication of the central tendency, and tends to underestimate the population range. The maximum is often used to mislead, particularly in advertising. The phrase "up

Table 3.5 Calculating the range

ID	Annual salary (£)
8	9,000
1	12,000
3	12,000
7	12,500
2	13,000
6	13,000
9	13,500
5	15,000
10	24,000
4	100,000

to" allows strong claims to be made about products. A shampoo that offers "up to 70 per cent less breakage", is reporting the maximum or best possible improvement, giving no indication of the central tendency or range of values, for that matter. Put differently, it is only telling part of the story.

Box 3.3 R code to calculate the range

```
range(x) #provides the range of a variable x
```

Interquartile range

The interquartile range is the middle half of the data, or the middle 50 per cent. To calculate the interquartile range, first calculate quartile 1 (Q1), the first quarter. Then calculate the third quartile (Q3). Subtracting Q1 from Q3 gives the interquartile range. A quick method is to divide the sorted values in half, and then find the median in each half. The median of the first half is the first quartile. The median of the second half is the third quartile. If you have a data set with an odd sample size, include its median in both halves.

Box 3.4 R code to calculate quartiles

```
quartile(x) # gives the quartiles of x: 0%, 25%, 50%, 75%
# and 100%
```

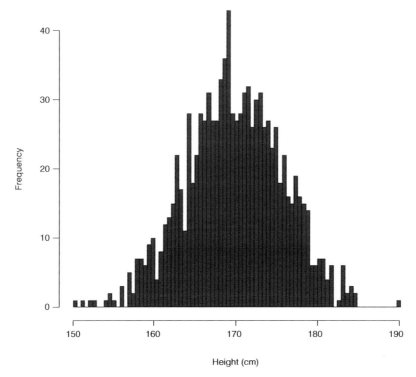

Figure 3.1 Normal distribution

The normal distribution

The graph in Figure 3.1 is a frequency histogram. This frequency histogram shows a larger sample of heights taken from the population. Histograms are used for continuous variables. Unlike bar charts, used for categorical variables, there are no gaps between the bars. This can be a helpful way to identify what kind of variable is being shown.

This distribution is normally distributed, having a bell-shaped curve. When data are normally distributed, the mean, median and mode are usually found in the same place. The mode can easily be identified as the tallest bar in a histogram, representing the most popular value.

Box 3.5 R code for normal distributions

```
x<-rnorm(1000, mean = 100, sd = 15) #generates a normal
# distribution for a sample size of 1000, having a mean of 100
# and standard deviation of 15. Recall that x<- means "x is"
hist(x) #shows a histogram of the data you generated,
# illustrating a normal distribution
```

Other kinds of distributions

Figure 3.2 shows kinds of distribution. Many variables are normally distributed, such as height, weight or blood pressure (top panel). We saw that when data are normally distributed, the mean, median and mode are in the same place. However, the distribution in the middle panel is skewed to the left. This is negative skew, because there is a build-up of negative values, leaving a longer tail toward the right. When data are skewed to the right (lower panel), this is called positive skew. The median is the best measure of central tendency for these types of distributions, because it better represents where the true central tendency lies.

The main point here is that you should always consider the distribution of your data before deciding what the best model of central tendency should be. For data which are not normally distributed, you can report the

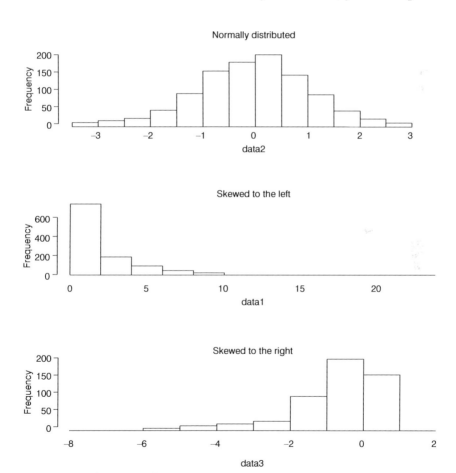

Figure 3.2 Kinds of distribution

Box 3.6 R code for generating skewed and normal distributions

```
data1<-exp(rnorm(1000,0,1))
data2<-rnorm(1000,0,1)
data3<-log(rnorm(1000,0,1))
par(mfrow=c(3,1))
hist(data1, main="Normally distributed")
hist(data2, main="Skewed to the left")
hist(data3, main="Skewed to the right")
new<-data.frame(data1,data2,data3)
write.table(new, file = "mydata.csv", sep = ",", col.names =
NA)
```

Box 3.7 R code for summarising variables

After loading in the heights data, you can request a summary of your variable(s) by using summary(x) where x is the name of the variable.

```
data <- read.table('height.csv', header=TRUE, sep=',')
attach(data)
summary(height)
```

---

median and interquartile range. Alternatively, you can report the five-point summary. This is the minimum, first quartile, the median, the third quartile and the maximum [3]. You could also consider transforming the data (see the section on 'Transformations' below). A simple way to obtain several different measures of central tendency for your data is to use the summary function in R, shown in Box3.7

Measures of dispersion

Error

The mean is only part of the story data have to tell. The histograms in Figure 3.3 show the frequency of different heights in two populations. Both populations have the same mean height, which is 168cm. They also have the same sample size, which is 10,000. In both cases, the mean is simpler than the data. It also makes full use of the available data, providing a model that is one piece of information – rather than 10,000 separate values. However, it hides two very different patterns. Data 2 is more spread out, in other words, more dispersed. To tell the two stories, we need another model. The second model needs to communicate the dispersion around the mean. It needs to accompany the mean – in fact we would always report measures of central tendency and dispersion together. This will complete the story, while still providing a useful

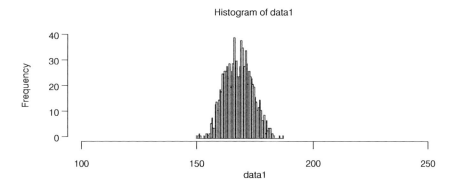

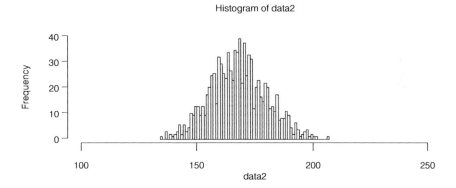

Figure 3.3 Different distributions

model that describes the mean and the dispersion using just two pieces of information.

A measure of dispersion needs to communicate an important pattern in the data. How 'spread out' are the data? How dispersed are the data? We want to model the variability in the data, but variability from what? The answer is variability from the mean. The mean is a centre of a normal distribution and we need to know how variable the data are from this point. How far away is each height from the mean height? In other words, what is the variance between the model of everyone's heights, and the raw data? This is called the error. How much error is there between the model and the data?

To find out how much error there is, we can subtract the mean from the raw data. The mean is the model, so this calculation will tell us the difference between the model and the data, which is the error. The error is also called the residual, meaning 'left over', or deviation, meaning deviation from the mean. If we add up (sum) the error, this should tell us the total amount of deviation from the mean (Table 3.6).

Table 3.6 Calculating error

ID	Height (cm)	Subtract mean	Error
1	168.7	167.97	0.73
2	172.0	167.97	4.03
3	176.5	167.97	8.53
4	160.5	167.97	–7.47
5	174.0	167.97	6.03
6	168.6	167.97	0.63
7	160.0	167.97	–7.97
8	163.0	167.97	–4.97
9	175.0	167.97	7.03
10	161.4	167.97	–6.57
		Sum	0

Variance

The answer we obtained was zero, so why did this strategy not work? It is clearly not true that there is no error between the model and the data. The sum of deviations from the mean is zero, but this does not mean that the data deviated from the mean. The answer is because of the direction of these deviations – some deviances are positive and some are negative. A solution is simply to square the deviances from the mean. Squaring values means we can ignore the direction of the errors, while still modelling their size. This is because the square of a negative number is a positive number. Calculating the sum of square errors gives 362.90, which should be divided by the sample size minus 1. This is the variance (Table 3.7).

We have calculated the variance of the height data, which is 40.32 cm^2. Is the variance a good model? It is clearly simpler than the data. It also makes the most of the data, if we acknowledge that we have used up a degree of freedom (see the section of degrees of freedom below). It does tell the right story – that the average error in the data is 40.32 cm^2. However, this is not very appealing for the audience. It is better to convert this back into centimetres, by taking the square root of the variance. This is the standard deviation (SD), described below.

Box 3.8 R code for variance

Use var(x) where x is the variable name. For example:

```
var(height)
```

Table 3.7 Calculating variance and standard deviation

ID	Height (cm)	Subtract mean	Error	Squared error
1	168.7	−167.97	0.73	0.53
2	172.0	−167.97	4.03	16.24
3	176.5	−167.97	8.53	72.76
4	160.5	−167.97	−7.47	55.80
5	174.0	−167.97	6.03	36.36
6	168.6	−167.97	0.63	0.40
7	160.0	−167.97	−7.97	63.52
8	163.0	−167.97	−4.97	24.70
9	175.0	−167.97	7.03	49.42
10	161.4	−167.97	−6.57	43.16

$$s^2 = \frac{\sum (x - \bar{x})^2}{(n-1)}$$

Sum of squared errors	362.90
Variance	40.32
Standard deviation	6.35cm

Standard deviation

The standard deviation is calculated by taking the square root of the variance:

$$SD = \sqrt{s^2}$$

The sample standard deviation s, estimates the population standard deviation – just as the sample mean estimates the population mean. Larger standard deviations suggest that there is more dispersion, or variability. Smaller standard deviations suggest that there is less dispersion or variability. The mean and standard deviation are descriptive statistics and should be reported together. Taken together, are they good models? They are more simple than the data. In our example, they describe ten pieces of information using two values. They make the most of the data, because all of the data is

---

Box 3.9 An aside: converting standard errors to standard deviations

You can convert standard errors (SE) to standard deviations, and vice versa, using the following formulae:

$$SE = \frac{SD}{\sqrt{n}}$$

$$SD = SE \times \sqrt{n}$$

This is sometimes helpful to know, because you might have access to the standard error but not the standard deviation, or vice versa, particularly when appraising other people's research (Chapters 7 to 11).

---

used in the calculation. They also communicate a *better* story than the mean alone. They model the central tendency *and* spread.

Remember that the purpose of modelling data is to simplify it by communicating its important features to a specified audience. We can communicate three important features of this data using just three values (mean, standard deviation and *n*). When reporting the mean and standard deviation and working by hand, remember these four rules:

1 Work to four decimal places.

2 Round up or down at the last step, remembering that values of 5 or greater should be rounded up.

3 Avoid what has been called 'pseudo-precision' [3]. If the data are measured at one decimal place, there is no point in reporting at two or more decimal places. There is no added value in reporting height at two decimal places, if it was recorded to the nearest centimetre.

4 Always report the mean and standard deviation together, with the units and the sample size.

Box 3.10 R code for standard deviation

Use sd(x) where x is the variable name. For example:

```
sd(height) #note that sd function is R uses the denominator
# n-1, as in this chapter
```

Degrees of freedom

The equation for the variance shows that we divide by the sample size minus 1, not by the sample size. This happens because we only have one degree of freedom left, when reaching nine of the ten deviations in the table (or in any sample, $n-1$ degrees of freedom). Once we have calculated nine, the remaining one can be calculated from all the others because they all add to zero. For this reason, only nine of the ten deviations are independent from each other, a situation described as having nine degrees of freedom. It has been shown that dividing by $n-1$ rather than n better estimates the variance in the population [20]. Be careful when using Excel however, because there is more than one way to calculate the standard deviation =STDEV.P(A1:A10) and =STDEV.S(A1:A10). It is recommended that you use STDEV.S since this uses $n-1$, which provides a better result because it acknowledges that the data are from a sample, not a population. The terminology is slightly confusing, because we might think that STDEV.S would be the appropriate command to use when working with a sample. In fact, it means standard deviation *of* a sample.

> **Box 3.11** R code for a summary of central tendency and dispersion
>
> The sample size, mean, median and standard deviation for any variable can be obtained in the epibasix package using the function univar(x) where x is the name of the variable. For example:
>
> ```
> require(epibasix) #you may need to install the epibasix
> # package if not already available
> univar(height)
> ```

Standard error

We know that larger samples estimate the mean more precisely than smaller samples. But how much more precisely? We can model precision using a statistic. It is called the standard error of the mean. You might say, 'we don't know what the population mean is – how can we possibly model how precisely it is measured?' Well, we can estimate precision by using the sample standard deviation and the sample size. The following section will explain how this is achieved.

Sampling distribution of the mean

The reason why we take samples from a population is because we want to estimate what the value might be in that population. Table 3.8 shows the notation used to distinguish sample from population statistics for mean and standard deviation. It is important to use the correct notation, to be sure that we know which statistic we are talking about. We can calculate the mean and standard deviation in our sample, but rarely do we know the mean and standard deviation in the population. We hope that the mean and standard deviation in our sample are close to what they would be in the population, but how close are they? How much margin of error is there? In turns out that although the population mean cannot be known, the sample standard deviation can be used to estimate the population standard deviation. This is extremely useful because it allows us to calculate a standard error of the mean, used to construct confidence intervals (CIs) around the sample mean.

   Suppose that we took many, many different samples from a population. We could calculate many different means from these samples. These could be plotted in a histogram. This frequency distribution of all the different means is called the sampling distribution (of means). It is a hypothetical distribution

Table 3.8 Sample notation

	Mean	Standard deviation
Sample	$\bar{x}$	s
Population	μ	σ

of all possible means from all possible samples of the same size, from the same population. The sampling distribution has three important and useful features:

1 it is normal, if the data are normally distributed in the population;

2 its mean is the same as the population mean;

3 its standard deviation can be used to show how precisely the sample mean estimates the population mean.

These three facts have been established previously and can be shown to be true in simulation studies. The book website contains a link to a simulation demonstration on the web, where you can explore these assumptions in more detail. For now, we can use these facts to calculate a statistic called the standard error of the sample mean. The standard error of the sample mean is the statistic used to show how precisely the sample mean estimates the population mean.

$$\text{SE} = s / \sqrt{n}$$

Larger standard errors indicate that the sample mean estimates the population mean less precisely. Smaller standard errors indicate the sample mean estimates the population more precisely. The standard deviation in our sample tells us something about the variability in the population, and therefore how precisely we are likely to have estimated the population mean. The sample standard deviation, then, provides a linkage between the sample and the population. The standard deviation in the sample becomes a proxy for the standard deviation in the population.

In this equation, you can see that the standard deviation of the sample is adjusted for the (square root of) the sample size. Larger samples, then, produce smaller standard errors. They estimate the mean more precisely. You can also see that the standard error depends on the variation in the population. If the population has less variation, the sample standard deviation we obtain would be smaller, and so would the standard error.

Z-scores

Z-scores refer to the normal distribution expressed in standardised units (mean = 0, standard deviation = 1). This means that a z-score of 1 is one standard deviation (SD) above the mean, and a z-score of –1 is one SD below the mean. It is also helpful to know that one standard deviation covers 68 percent of values, two standard deviations cover 95 per cent and three cover 99.7 per cent. For example, the SF-36 Physical and Mental Component Summaries (www.sf36.org) are often used as measures of self-reported health status. The scales have a mean of 50 and SD of 10. This means that:

- 68% of people will score 40 to 60;

- 95% of people will score 30 to 70;

- 99.7% of people will score 20 to 80.

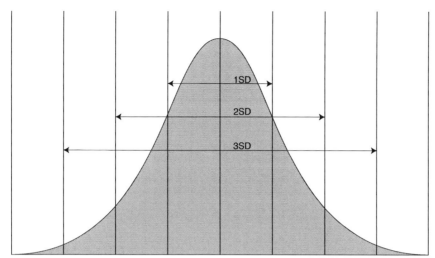

Figure 3.4 Standard deviations and coverage of population

T-scores

T-scores have a mean of 50 and a standard deviation of 10 (the SF-36 has a *T*-score scoring method). This can be more intuitively appealing than *z*-scores. Knowing that the mean is 50 can be easier to visualise than a mean of 10. The range for *T*-scores, however, is obscure. Although it conceptually ranges from 0 to 100, it is possible to have extremely low scores that are below 0 (negative) and above 100.

Confidence intervals for a mean

Once we know the mean and standard deviation of a variable in a sample, we can calculate confidence intervals around this estimate. Confidence intervals provide a range of plausible estimates for the population mean. They are often interpreted as meaning that there is a 95 per cent probability that the population mean is somewhere within their range. This is intuitively appealing, but incorrect. It is more accurate to say that if we kept taking samples from the same population, 95 per cent of the confidence intervals would be expected to contain the population mean [20]. This means that 1 in 20 studies (5 per cent) would produce confidence intervals that do not contain the population mean – a point worth remembering.

When the sample size is small the assumption that the data are normally distributed is often violated. This means that you should use the *t*-distribution rather than the *z*-distribution to calculate the confidence interval (see *z*-tables in Appendix 3 and *t*-tables in Appendix 1). Historically, different cut-points for determining 'large' sample sizes have been advocated. Traditionally, a *t*-value has been used to create confidence intervals around the mean for a small sample, a *z*-value for large samples. This was necessary when working by hand with a calculator. Most of the time in practice, we use statistical software to compute the *p*-value, and this distinction between 'small' and 'large' is perhaps unnecessary.

$x \pm (t \cdot SE)$

Example: Confidence interval for the mean (small sample)

The BMI values for ten patients undergoing spinal surgery was recorded by a nurse. Calculate the confidence intervals for the mean in the population (all candidates for spinal surgery).

When the sample size is large, use the *z* formula:

$x \pm (z \cdot SE)$

Table 3.9 Confidence interval for the mean (small sample)

ID	BMI	Subtract mean	Error	Squared error
1	30	−26.7	3.3	10.89
2	22	−26.7	−4.7	22.09
3	27	−26.7	0.3	0.09
4	30	−26.7	3.3	10.89
5	25	−26.7	−1.7	2.89
6	28	−26.7	1.3	1.69
7	21	−26.7	−5.7	32.49
8	22	−26.7	−4.7	22.09
9	29	−26.7	2.3	5.29
10	33	−26.7	6.3	39.69

Calculating the 95% confidence interval for the mean	Sum of squared errors	148.1
SE = 4.06 / 9 = 1.35	Variance	16.46
Lower interval = 26.7 − (1.96×1.35) = 24.05	SD	4.06
Upper interval = 26.7 + (1.96×1.35) = 29.35	SE	1.35
How this should be reported:	Lower	24.05
The mean BMI was 26.7 (95%CI 24.05 to 29.35)	Upper	29.35

Box 3.12 Exercise: Confidence interval for the mean (large sample)

Suppose that the mean (SD) forced expiratory volume in one second (FEV_1) is 2.97 (0.78) litres in a sample of 6735 adults from the general population. Assuming that the sample is representative of the population, what is the 95% CI for the mean FEV_1 value?

$$SE = \frac{0.78}{\sqrt{6734}} = 0.0095$$

Lower interval = 2.97 − (1.96 × 0.0095) = 2.9514

Upper interval = 2.97 + (1.96 × 0.0095) = 2.9886

How this could be reported:

The mean FEV_1 value was 2.97 (95% CI 2.95 to 2.99) litres.

In this example, I would suggest working with the standard error at four significant figures and reporting the confidence intervals to four decimal places.

You can also calculate 99% confidence intervals, by using the value of 3.72 from the z distribution. This is less commonly done, but is perfectly valid:

Lower interval = 2.97 − (3.72 × 0.0095) = 2.9347

Upper interval = 2.97 + (3.72 × 0.0095) = 3.0053

How this could be reported:

The mean FEV_1 value was 2.97 (99% CI 2.94 to 3.00) litres.

The 99% confidence intervals are wider, but not much wider, in this example.

There is clearly no need to take a sample of 6735 people from the population in order to estimate the mean FEV1 value in the population. A smaller sample would produce a reasonably narrow 95% confidence interval. But how small? Choice of sample size is governed by a formal sample size calculation, discussed in Appendix 7.

Comparing the mean to a known value

It may be useful to compare a sample mean to a known value. For example, suppose that we are conducting a research study in which height might be an important variable to consider. The research assistant has been asked to display a poster advertising the study in the student union building. Unfortunately, he places it below the area on the notice board reserved for the male basketball team. The professor is now worried that tall males are more likely to become over-represented in the study, and the sample is therefore not representative. He has asked you to find out if it differs significantly from the population value. *The Health Survey for England* (2008) data provide the population mean height (175.3, SE = 0.11) for males [21]. Our sample (n = 30) has a mean height of 175.9 (SE = 2.00) and we are concerned that they are slightly taller than the general population. Notice how much larger the standard error is here – the sample is only 30 people. Does the height in our sample differ significantly from population height? In order to determine this, we need to find out how far away our sample mean is from the population mean.

$$z = \frac{(x - \mu_0)}{(s / \sqrt{n})}$$

This formula assumes that the variable (height) is continuous and normally distributed.

$$z = (175.9 - 175.3)/2.00 = 0.30$$

The z-value of 0.30 tells us that the mean difference is 0.3 standard errors away from zero (the null value). We can obtain the probability of getting a mean difference of this size from the z-table. The first decimal place is 3, the second is 0. The probability shown in the cell is 0.3085. This is greater than the value of 0.05 traditionally adopted as the threshold for statistical significance. Therefore, the null hypothesis that any difference between the mean is due to chance, is retained. The data we observed are not statistically significantly different from the population. In this example, this could mitigate concerns that the individuals in the sample are taller than the population. They might be unrepresentative in other ways, however, and you might have concerns that sampling from student union buildings will lead to bias. These kinds of issues are considered in the critical appraisal chapters. For now, our main concern is the difference in means.

You might also have concerns that the sample is too small. As mentioned previously in the exercise and in Appendix 7, sample size should ideally be determined using a formal sample size calculation. Assuming that 30 people is sufficient for this study and is the final sample available, our main problem is that the data are not normally distributed. In this situation you can use the t-statistic, unless the data are severely non-normal and should be transformed or ranked (see separate sections on 'Transformations' and 'Ranked data' on these topics).

$$t = \frac{(x - \mu_0)}{(s/\sqrt{n})}, \qquad d.f. = 1$$

$t = (175.9 - 175.3)/2.00 = 0.30$ (29 degrees of freedom)

The t-table involves a different method to the z-table. First locate the appropriate number of degrees of freedom (29) then the level of statistical significance required. This is usually 0.05 and a two-sided p-value, if we did not make a prediction about which *direction* the means would differ in. Since we hypothesised that our sample would be taller, a one-sided test is required. The appropriate cell indicates that a value of 1.70. This is the value of t that would be required in order to reject the null hypothesis that any difference in means is due to chance. Our value is smaller than 1.70 at 0.30, again suggesting that the difference we observed is due to chance.

Certainty or precision?

It may be helpful to calculate 99 per cent confidence intervals rather than 95 per cent confidence intervals. A 99 per cent confidence interval obviously has greater certainty, capturing a wider range of plausible values for the population mean. On the other hand, a 99 per cent interval is necessarily wider than a 95 per cent interval, and so is less precise. This shows that there is always a trade-

Table 3.10 z-values and confidence intervals

Length of interval	z-value
68%	0.99
95%	1.96
99%	2.58

off between certainty and precision, when choosing the size of a confidence interval to use. The convention is to use 95 per cent confidence intervals, although this is somewhat arbitrary. The z-value of 1.96 is the 5 percentage point of the normal distribution: 95 per cent of distribution lies between –1.96 and 1.96. Table 3.10 shows different z-values that can be used to change the width of confidence intervals, to some popular alternatives.

Transformations

Many variables are measured on scales which produce negatively or positively skewed distributions (see section of 'Other types of distribution'). Examples include C-reactive protein (a measure of inflammation), salivary cortisol (often used as a marker of sensitivity to psychosocial stressors) and incomes (because there is a small number of people with very high incomes). Reporting the median, a measure of central tendency described above, is one solution. When attempting to describe the standard deviation however, particularly in several different groups, skewed data can produce misleading results. Transformations are another possible solution.

When data are positively or negatively skewed, it can sometimes be useful to transform them onto a different scale. Changing the scale does not change the data itself, but it does change the relative distance between each point on the scale. A familiar example is the Richter earthquake magnitude scale, which communicates the strength of earthquakes. A magnitude of less than 2 is so small that people do not generally notice the quake. Earthquakes with a score of 4 would shake and rattle indoor objects. A score of 7 would cause serious damage over a large area. Extremely large earthquakes are much more powerful than is implied by the Richter scale, if we misinterpreted to imply equal distances between each value. You might think that the transformed scale has the same distance between 1 and 2 as between 7 and 8, but this is not correct. Transformations are useful because they compress large values, bringing the tail of the distribution inwards. They also have the additional advantage of decompressing smaller values.

Logarithms to the base 10 transform data so that the difference between 1 and 10 becomes the same as the distance between 10 and 100, 1,000 and 10,000, and so on. The principle is exactly the same as for the Richter scale, producing a new scale that is easier to visualise and therefore more intuitive. As shown in Table 3.10, the distance between 1 and 2 is the same as the distance between 9 and 10, when using the transformed scale. The transformation is achieved using the following formula:

Table 3.11 Logarithmic scales

ID	x	log10(x)
1	−1	Not possible
2	0	Not possible
3	1	0
4	10	1
5	100	2
6	1000	3
7	10000	4
8	100000	5
9	1000000	6
10	10000000	7

$$x = 10^u = \log 10(x)$$

For example:
$$1000000 = 10 \times 10 \times 10 \times 10 \times 10 \times 10 = 10^6 = \log 10(6)$$

Put differently, this means that the logarithm to base 10 of 6 (log10(6)) is the same as ten to the power of six, or ten times ten six times. So if we were told that someone had a score of 6 on a logarithmic scale (having base 10), we would know that this actually means their true score was 1000000 (see Table 3.11). We can take the antilog (10^x) to reverse the transformation, since 10^6 is 1000000. In Excel and R, this is achieved by using `10^x`.

$$10^6 = 1000000$$

Distributions with very large numbers can therefore be converted into more manageable numbers.

Box 3.13 An aside: a war magnitude scale

Lewis Fry Richardson was a statistician put in charge of organising data on war causalities [22]. Since a terrorist campaign might involve around 100 casualties, but larger wars might involve over 1 million, he decided that the data were suitable for logarithmic transformation. He proposed that logarithmic to base 10 could be used to classify wars. A terror campaign resulting in 100 deaths would receive a score of 2, a war with 1 million deaths a score of 6, and so on. The Vietnam War, for example, would receive a score of 4.7 (around 50,000 deaths). This war magnitude scale is psychologically helpful, because people can more easily interpret the impact of human violence on one scale [22], since larger numbers are often harder to visualise.

Table 3.12 C-reactive protein (CRP)data

ID	CRP	ln(CRP)
1	2.718282	1
2	7.389056	2
3	20.08554	3
4	54.59815	4
5	148.4132	5
6	403.4288	6
7	1096.633	7
8	2980.958	8
9	8103.084	9
10	22026.47	10

Note that log transformations are not permissible on negative values or on zero. Sometimes a constant is added to all the data values to get around this problem, typically one, to make all the values positive. If so, this should be reported when describing results. It may be necessary to remove the constant, particularly when transforming data back to the original scale (back transforming).

It is more common to use the natural logarithm, rather than base ten. The natural logarithm uses a mathematical constant called e, but the principle is the same as for base ten. The value of e is 2.7182818 for reasons which are not important here, and e is usually built into most calculators so that it can be used automatically.

$$403.4288 = e \times e \times e \times e \times e \times e = e^6$$

$$e^6 = 403.4288$$

To illustrate, we will look at some data on C-reactive protein (CRP), which is a measure of inflammation (Table 3.12). The distribution is positively skewed, having a long tail to the right. Taking the natural logarithm of these values produces something closer to a normal distribution (middle column). With only 10 values, we would not expect to see a perfectly symmetrical bell shaped curve, but we have improved the distribution. For checking purposes, we can take the antilog, which returns the values back to their original scale (right hand column). CRP can be said to have a lognormal distribution, because it is normal when shown on the log scale. The natural logarithm uses base e, a mathematical constant often used in a variety of situations.

Many people find logarithms to base 10 easier to understand than the natural logarithm. Many statistical methods and software packages use the natural logarithm, however, and so this is used throughout this book. Logistic regression, for example, requires that you understand how to take the exponent (antilog) for values which are presented on a natural logarithm scale.

Here is a summary of reasons why we might want to transform data:

- associations between the skewed variable and other variables will not appear to be linear, when in fact they might be;

- people find logarithmic scales easier to visualise (e.g. the Richter scale) and understand;

- standard deviations in different groups could be very different;

- logistic regression produces results which are on a natural logarithmic scale (Chapter 14).

Summary

In this chapter several statistics have been introduced. Some are measures of central tendency (mean, median, mode, range). Some are measures of dispersion (error, standard error, variance, standard deviation). Two approaches to statistical analysis have also been introduced: methods of estimation (confidence intervals) and hypothesis testing (p-values). Remember that the variance is the average squared distance from the mean divided by n–1. The standard deviation is the square root of the variance, and is therefore a measure of dispersion using the same units as the original observations. The standard deviation qualifies the mean, and is essential to report alongside it (when the mean is the best measure of central tendency). If data are skewed, the median is the best measure of central tendency. Qualify the median by also reporting the five-point summary.

## 4

Measures of association for categorical outcomes

The chapter will demonstrate how to differentiate risk and odds and how to decide which is a more appropriate method to use in a particular context. When diseases are common, the risk and odds could provide seemingly very different information, and this chapter will show you how to calculate them in ways that help you to estimate the probability of an event happening. The chapter uses the example of smokers and non-smokers to demonstrate how to calculate the risk of lung cancer among smokers. It also shows you how to calculate the risk difference, attributable risk or excess risk; this is the difference in risk between the exposed and unexposed group.

The chapter builds on this by showing you how to calculate the number needed to treat (NNT) and the number needed to harm (NNH). These statistics tell you how many patients would have to receive an exposure, in order to prevent or produce a single case of the disease. It also helps you to differentiate between the individual and the population. This is a useful way to inform cost-effectiveness calculations in, for example, public health interventions such as smoking cessation campaigns. The chapter then demonstrates how to calculate relative measures of risk, which communicate the population view and therefore also usefully informs public health intervention decisions.

Researchers often need to gather data using a variety of methodologies, including postal questionnaires. The chapter includes an exercise which uses relative risk calculation to help you to maximise the response rate for postal questionnaires during research. The chapter then discusses odds ratios, a way of working out the odds of a disease developing based on an exposure when using a case control study, which means we cannot calculate the relative risk. The odds ratio approximates the relative risk in this case. Odds ratios are also useful as they are used to adjust for confounding factors in statistical models which take into account more than two variables.

The chapter closes with an exercise enabling you to test your understanding of absolute versus relative risk. In practical terms, this allows you to work out the value of prescribing a new drug, both in terms of the efficacy of the drug and the cost of preventing the disease.

Introduction

A great deal of health research is concerned with outcomes which are categorical. Is a disease present or not? Did the patient die, or are they still alive? Did the event occur, or has it not occurred? Similarly, we are often concerned with relationship of a health outcome to an exposure. Exposures are frequently categorical. Was someone exposed or not exposed? Did the patient receive the treatment, or not? Which people smoked and which did not smoke? This chapter introduces measures of association for categorical outcomes, and we will focus on situations in which an exposure is also categorical. The term 'exposure' is a general one, referring to variables that can be either protective or harmful. For example, an exposure could be a risk factor in the environment, or a new drug intended to reduce the risk of a disease occurring.

Intended learning outcomes

By the end of this chapter, you should be able to define, calculate and interpret:

- risk and odds
- absolute measures of risk
- relative measures of risk
- number needed to treat and number needed to harm
- simple tabular data from published research studies.

Calculations will be performed by hand, and also in R. Throughout this chapter, we will use the generalised notation for two-by-two contingency tables, shown in Table 4.1. The outcome is categorical and binary, meaning that it can only take two values. For example, the outcome might be disease or healthy, event or non-event. We will also be working with exposures that are categorical. For example, exposed or unexposed, smoker or non-smoker, treatment or control. For these kinds of examples, people in the study can only belong to one of four cells. They can either be exposed or unexposed, diseased or healthy.

Table 4.1 Generalized notation for 2 × 2 tables in this book

	Disease	*Healthy*	*Total*
Exposed	a	b	e
Unexposed	c	d	f
Total	g	h	*N*

Risk and odds

Risk

Risk concerns the chance that something will happen, in relation to the chance that everything will happen. The term 'risk' is synonymous with the term 'probability'. Probability is a continuous variable, ranging from 0 to 1. The zero is a true zero, and this would mean that there is no chance of the event occurring. The one is the maximum number available, meaning that the event definitely will happen. The risk that a disease will occur has to lie between 0 and 1. For example, suppose that the risk of dying from heart disease is 0.2 or 20 per cent. This is the same as saying that 1 in 5 people die from heart disease.

$$\text{risk} = \frac{1}{5} = 0.2 = 20\%$$

Risk always lies between 0 and 1, or equivalently, between 0 and 100%.

Odds

Odds concerns the chance that something will happen, in relation to the chance that something will not happen. Odds are slightly less intuitive than risks, because most people tend to prefer thinking about chance as a probability. People who bet on horses tend to be more familiar with odds. To illustrate the odds of something happening, take the example of heart disease. Death from heart disease occurs in one person to every four people who do not die from heart disease. Therefore, the odds are 1 to 4, or 0.25.

$$\text{odds} = \frac{1}{4} = 0.25 = 25\%$$

Odds can range from 0 to infinity, moving above 1 if the event is more common than the non-event. This is usually not encountered in the health sciences, where we tend to study disease outcomes that are less common than non-disease outcomes. Odds are a different way of communicating the chance of the same event. We can choose to calculate the risk or the odds. However, risks and odds often take different values. In the heart disease example, the risk is 0.2 and the odds are 0.25. These appear, at first reading, to communicate quite different things. Neither is necessarily a better or more accurate way of communicating the chance of dying of heart disease, providing that we are clear what the number refers to. Why then, do health scientists need to use two different ways of communicating chance? Why not focus on risks, since they are more intuitively meaningful? The short answer is, that both risks and odds have specific advantages, in different contexts. A longer answer is provided later on in this chapter and in the chapter on logistic regression.

Table 4.2 illustrates the risk and odds for a range of 'everyday' events [23]. What do you notice about the risk and odds, as you move down the table?

You should notice that the risk and odds are different for common events, such as heart disease, but gradually become more similar. We can see that risk and odds are generally the same, but only for rare events. This is worth bearing

Table 4.2 Familiar events expressed as risk and odds

	Chance expressed as risk	_Risk_	_Chance expressed as odds_	_Odds_
Dying from heart disease	1 in 5	0.2000000	1 to 4	0.2500000
Dying from cancer	1 in 7	0.1428571	1 to 6	0.1666667
Getting three balls in the UK national lottery	1 in 11	0.0909091	1 to 10	0.1000000
Transmission of measles	1 in 100	0.0100000	1 to 99	0.0101010
Annual risk of death, smoking 10 per day	1 in 200	0.0050000	1 to 199	0.0050251
Death by air travel incident	1 in 20 000	0.0000500	1 to 19 999	0.0000500
Death playing football	1 in 50 000	0.0000200	1 to 49 999	0.0000200
Death by murder	1 in 100 000	0.0000100	1 to 99 999	0.0000100
Death by rail accident	1 in 500 000	0.0000020	1 to 499 999	0.0000020
Drowning in the bath in the next year	1 in 685 000	0.0000015	1 to 684 999	0.0000015
Getting six balls in the UK national lottery	1 in 2 796 763	0.0000004	1 to 2 796 762	0.0000004
Death from a nuclear power accident	1 in 10 000 000	0.0000001	1 to 9 999 999	0.0000001

Box 4.1 An aside: odds and risk

Odds are commonly used by gamblers in betting shops. Suppose that the odds of Barking Football Club winning the cup are 10 to 1. This means that the bookmaker thinks the chance of Barking not winning are ten times the chance that they will. Put different, for every time that the team will win, they will lose 10 times. Counter-intuitively, bookmakers normally express the likelihood of the non-event (10), compared to the event (1). Therefore, the odds are 0.1 in this scenario. Most people are more familiar with the probability (risk) of an event. Fortunately, we can easily convert odds to risk, and vice versa.

$$\text{odds} = \frac{\text{risk}}{1 - \text{risk}} = \frac{0.1}{1 - 0.1} = 0.11$$

$$\text{risk} = \frac{\text{odds}}{1 + \text{odds}} = \frac{0.11}{1 + 0.11} = 0.1$$

In this example, the odds and risk are fairly similar. This is because the outcome is relatively rare.

in mind because it will become important later. When diseases are common, the risk and odds could provide seemingly very different information. *Odds tend to over-estimate the chance that something happens, when the event is common.* For rare diseases, it doesn't often matter whether we use risk or odds. However, most researchers tend to use odds, for varieties of reasons, which are discussed below.

Calculating absolute risk

Measures of absolute risk tell us what the chance is that an event happens, taking into account all of the possible events. Put differently, what is the chance that an event happens, out of the chance that everything happens? In this hypothetical data [20] (Table 4.3), we are shown the incidence of lung cancer after one year, following recruitment into a prospective cohort study. What is the chance (risk) of lung cancer among smokers?

Table 4.3 Risk of lung cancer among smokers

	Lung cancer one year later	Healthy	Total
Smoker	39	29 961	30 000
Non-smoker	6	59 994	60 000
Total	45	89 955	90 000

Calculating the proportion of disease cases in the exposed group

To calculate the risk of lung cancer among smokers, we want to know the proportion of cases of lung cancer among the exposed group. That is, the risk of lung cancer in the exposed group. This can be done by calculating the proportion of those with the disease in the exposed group (p_1), who developed lung cancer (see equation below). To calculate the proportion exposed, we divide 39 (the number of people with the disease who were exposed) by 30 000 (the total number of people exposed). This gives a proportion of 0.0013, or 0.13 per cent. This is the absolute risk of lung cancer among the exposed group. They have a 0.13% chance of developing lung cancer one year later.

$$p_1 = \frac{a}{e} = \frac{39}{30000} = 0.0013 = 0.13\%$$

Risk difference, or attributable risk

The risk difference is the difference in risk between the exposed group and the unexposed group. To calculate the risk difference, we need to work out the proportion of people with the disease among the unexposed group (p_0), and then subtract this from the proportion in the exposed group. Dividing 6 (the number of people with the disease who were unexposed) by 60 000 (the total number of people unexposed) gives a proportion of 0.0001 or 0.01 per cent.

$$p_0 = \frac{a}{f} = \frac{6}{60000} = 0.0001 = 0.01\%$$

The absolute risk difference is simply the difference between the two risks. It is sometimes called the 'attributable risk' or 'excess risk', meaning the proportion of extra risk which is accounted for by the exposure. Depending on the sign of the answer, the risk difference could refer to an absolute risk increase, or an absolute risk reduction (RD).

$$RD = p_1 - p_0 = 0.0013 - 0.001 = 0.0012$$

There is a proportion of 0.0012 or 0.12 per cent difference between the two groups. The risk among those exposed is higher, an absolute risk increase of 0.12 per cent. This seems rather small, but remember, that this is the excess risk for one individual over a relatively short time frame. It does not tell us how many times more likely the disease is for smokers, compared to non-smokers. Nor does it tell us how many smokers would have to stop smoking, in order to prevent one case. To work out these problems, we need to consider relative risks and the number needed to treat, which are introduced below. Additionally, if we wanted to work out the longer-term association between smoking and lung cancer over many years, a longer follow-up period would be necessary. This is not the focus of this chapter, concerned only with illustrative examples. Plenty of these kinds of studies have been conducted, reviewed elsewhere [24].

The risk difference is a useful starting point, but suppose that you wanted to calculate the impact of an exposure on your local community or a larger population. By impact, we mean the proportion of cases which are accounted for (and therefore preventable) by the exposure. To do that, we need to know what the prevalence of the disease in our population actually is. We can then simply subtract the rate of the disease in the population from the rate of disease in the unexposed group:

$$PAR = p_t - p_0 = \frac{g}{N} - \frac{c}{f} = \frac{45}{90000} - \frac{6}{60000} = 0.0005 - 0.0001 = 0.0004$$

It may be helpful to express this as a percentage of the cases which are attributable to the exposure. This is called the 'population attributable risk per cent' (PAR%). To calculate it, divide the PAR by the proportion with the disease in the population (p_t), then multiply by 100 to obtain the percentage:

$$PAR(\%) = 100\left(\frac{PAR}{A}\right) = 100\left(\frac{0.0004}{0.0005}\right) = 80\%$$

This indicates that 80 per cent of the risk of lung cancer during the follow-up period is attributable to smoking, according to the data provided. This estimate assumes that no other factors are involved, which is rarely the case, but for now we will assume that we have estimated the true association between smoking and lung cancer. If our assumption is correct, 80 per cent of cases of lung cancer might be preventable if we could remove this exposure from the environment. The other 20 per cent are due to other factors. The term 'population attributable risk' is used differently in different contexts, by different researchers, which can be confusing. For example, some people use the term 'attributable risk' to refer to the risk difference. Do not worry too much about differences in terminology. The key point to remember is that you should understand the difference between the absolute risk difference (which is simply the difference between two proportions) and the population attributable risk (which takes into account the prevalence of the disease in the population, and which can be expressed as a percentage). When appraising existing research, it should be clear from the context what the author is referring to. If it isn't clear, it may be possible to work it out for yourself, or ask the author for clarification.

Key points about absolute measures

- Absolute measures take into account the risk to an individual if they are not exposed.

- Absolute measures communicate the benefit to an individual of removing a risk factor or taking a treatment.

- Absolute risk measures can distinguish between small and large exposure

Number needed to treat (NNT) and number needed to harm (NNH)

The number needed to treat (NNT) and the number needed to harm (NNH) are useful statistics. They tell you how many patients would have to receive the exposure, in order to prevent or produce a single case of the disease. For example, a number needed to treat of 100 for a new drug tells us that 100 patients would have to be exposed to the new drug, in order to prevent one case. A number needed to harm of 50 for an exposure, means that 50 people would have to be exposed, to result in one case. The calculation for NNT is very simple. It is the reciprocal of the risk difference, which means the inverse of the risk difference, ignoring the sign. Put differently, we simply divide 1 by the size of the risk difference. Horizontal bars are used in equations, to indicate that we should ignore the sign. Returning to the example of smoking and lung cancer, we can calculate the NNH from the risk difference (rd) of 0.0012:

$$\text{NNH} = \frac{1}{|rd|} = \frac{1}{0.0012} = 833$$

This tells us that for every 833 smokers, 1 person would be expected to develop lung cancer one year later (rounded to the nearest whole person). This may surprise you, because we are used to thinking that smoking is a strong risk factor for lung cancer. However, it illustrates once again the importance of thinking about the bigger picture of population health.

- NNT is an intuitive way to think about absolute and relative risks, and the connection between them.

- Absolute measures communicate the clinical view. How many of your patients would have to receive the treatment, to prevent one case?

- NNT can be used to inform cost-effectiveness calculations.

Public health implications of NNT

From a public health perspective, it is worth encouraging 833 people not to start smoking (or 833 smokers to quit) so that one case of lung cancer can be prevented each year. From the perspective of an individual smoker, there may or may not be any meaningful reduction in risk associated with quitting. Many public health interventions are based on the premise that large numbers of people have to change their behaviour, in order to benefit the wider population, even if there is little benefit to those individuals in doing so. This is one reason why public health interventions are often unpopular with the general public. Why modify your lifestyle if there is little benefit to you as an individual? We return to this issue throughout the book. For now, just remember that there are always two sides to the story – the individual and the population. NNT is a useful and intuitive statistic for thinking about both, and is popular in clinical settings for this reason. Clinicians have to think about the benefit to individuals and their practice population.

Relative risk

The absolute risks from smoking, in the example above, seemed to be rather small. There is an absolute risk difference of just 0.12 per cent, an increase of 0.12 per cent for smokers. Absolute risk can tell us what the risk to the individuals exposed might be. The NNT can provide the clinical view, suggesting how many patients would have to be treated, to prevent one case. However, they can't tell us how many times more likely the exposed people are, than the unexposed, to develop a disease (the population view). To get this information, we need to know what the relative risk of the disease is, comparing the two groups. Relative risks are useful from the population perspective, because they take into account the fact that some outcomes are rare. Absolute risk differences can be small, but when we think of the bigger picture, the relative risk across the whole population might be cause for concern. This example will illustrate the difference between absolute and relative risks. So, we need to work out how many times more likely it is for the smokers to have lung cancer. That is, what is the relative risk of lung cancer, comparing those who smoked to those who did not? Relative risk (RR) is calculated by dividing the proportion exposed by the proportion unexposed:

$$\text{RR} = \frac{p_1}{p_0} = \frac{0.0013}{0.0001} = 13$$

This indicates that lung cancer after one year is 13 times more likely for smokers, than for non-smokers. Whereas the risk to an individual was an extra 0.0013 or 0.13 per cent, the risk when taking the population view is much larger. In Chapter 5, we will learn how to estimate how precisely this relative risk has been estimated, and whether or not it is statistically significant. For now, keep in mind that relative risks communicate a very different message about the association between smoking and lung cancer. The absolute risk increase and the relative risk are both accurate. They are simply two ways of communicating information about the size of the association. When deciding whether to communicate absolute or relative risks, your decision should be based on several different factors. These include the intended audience, the research question and whether the individual or population view is most appropriate. Very often, it is useful to calculate both the absolute and relative risk, particularly when conducting and reporting your own research.

Key points about relative measures of risk

- Relative risks are stable across different populations, even if those populations have different risks to begin with.

- Relative risks communicate the population view, which is important from a public health perspective.

- Relative risks do not tell us about the risk to individuals, and tend to overestimate the size of the effect. For this reason, drug companies and media may be choose to communicate the relative risk or relative risk reduction [25].

Exercise: Calculating a relative risk

Researchers are often keen to explore new ways of increasing the response rate for postal questionnaires. It has been suggested that a 'veiled threat' can make it more likely for people to return a postal questionnaire. A follow-up letter saying something along the lines of 'we have not yet received your questionnaire' contains a mild but implicit threat that further questionnaires will be sent, and that the respondent is being monitored. Table 4.4 shows some actual data from a randomised trial, which we can use to test this hypothesis [26]

Table 4.4 Postal questionnaire data

	Event (Returned questionnaire)	*Non-event (Did not return questionnaire)*	*Total*
Veiled threat	129	213	342
No threat	74	255	329
Total	203	468	671

Here, we have a slightly unusual situation in which the outcome is not a disease, but is a different kind of event – an event we want to happen. For this reason, the disease column has been relabelled as 'event', because the questionnaire coming back (the event) is the outcome we are interested in. The presence of a veiled threat does seem to increase the likelihood of the questionnaires coming back. We can probably determine this by scanning the data table, but we can calculate the relative risk to find out exactly how many times more likely it is. First, we calculate the proportion of responders in each group. Then we calculate the risk ratio.

$$p_1 = \frac{a}{e} = \frac{129}{342} = 0.3771$$

$$p_0 = \frac{a}{f} = \frac{74}{329} = 0.2249$$

$$RR = \frac{p_1}{p_0} = \frac{0.3771}{0.2249} = 1.68$$

The relative risk is 1.68, confirming our hypothesis that a veiled threat makes it more likely for a questionnaire to be returned (1.68 times more likely). We can see from the proportions that about 38 per cent of questionnaires are returned when a threat is present. About 23 per cent are returned even when no threat is present. If you decide to think about risks as percentages, it is important to distinguish percentages from percentage points. The risk difference is 0.1522, or 15.22 per cent (15.22 percentage points higher when a threat is present). The risk ratio suggests a 68 per cent increase in the probability of it being returned when a threat is included, compared to when it is not included.

Relative risk reduction

When the exposure has a protective effect, which is usually anticipated if the exposure is a treatment or intervention, it may be useful to calculate the relative risk reduction. This is the reduction in risk associated with having the treatment. For example, suppose that a new drug has an RR or 0.45 for reducing hospitalisation of children due to RSV infections (as shown in the real-life example below). We might want to calculate relative risk reduction (RRR) by:

$$RRR = 1 - RR = 1 - 0.45 = 0.55$$

This represents a relative risk reduction of 0.55 or 55 per cent.

Calculating 95% confidence intervals for the risk ratio

To calculate 95 per cent confidence intervals for the risk ratio (Table 4.5), first calculate the standard error of the RR on the log scale. Next, calculate an 'error factor' and then use this to calculate the lower and upper intervals. Finally, calculate the z-statistic to determine if the association is statistically significant (Chapter 2). The exact p-value can be obtained using R.

Table 4.5 Calculating CI for risk ratios

Maths notation	Example	In English
$SE \log RR = \sqrt{\dfrac{1}{a} - \dfrac{1}{e} + \dfrac{1}{c} - \dfrac{1}{f}}$	$SE \log RR = \sqrt{\dfrac{1}{129} - \dfrac{1}{342} + \dfrac{1}{74} - \dfrac{1}{329}}$ $= 0.123701096$	Take the reciprocal of cell a, subtract the reciprocal of cell e, add the reciprocal of cell c, subtract the reciprocal of cell f. Take the square root. This is the standard error of the log risk ratio.
$EF = \exp(1.96(SE \log RR))$	$EF = \exp(1.96 \times 0.1237)$ $= 1.2744$	Multiply the standard error of the log risk ratio by 1.96. Take the exponent of the answer, taking the result off the logarithmic scale. This is the error factor.
$95\% CI = \dfrac{RR}{EF},\ RR \times EF$	$= 1.68/1.2744,\ 1.68 \times 1.2744$ $= 1.3183,\ 2.1410$	To obtain the lower confidence interval, divide the risk ratio by the error factor. For the upper interval, multiply the risk ratio by the error factor.
$z = \dfrac{\log RR}{SE \log RR}$	$= 0.5188 / 0.1237$ $= 4.1940$ (1 d.f.)	To obtain the z-statistic, divide the natural log of the risk ratio by the standard error of the log risk ratio. Looking up the z-value in the table in the Appendix shows that the probability of the data under the null hypothesis is very small ($p < .01$).

Summary: Participants receiving a veiled threat were 1.68 times more likely to return the questionnaire (RR = 1.68, 95% CI 1.32 to 2.14, $p <.01$)

Table 4.6 Oesophageal cancer study data

	Oesophageal cancer	Healthy	Total
Exposed	65	30	95
Unexposed	235	570	805
Total	300	600	900

Odds ratios

Odds ratios are used to approximate the relative risk of a disease. They are very similar to the relative risk, when the disease is rare. You may wonder, then, why would we want to calculate an odds ratio? This is best illustrated with an example. The data in Table 4.6 is taken from a case control study, a type of study design which we will explore more fully in Chapter 10. Suppose that a researcher was interested in whether drinking steaming hot tea, rather than warm tea, increased the risk of oesophageal cancer [27].

We could work out what the absolute risk of the event (cancer) might be, for people who reported drinking steaming hot tea. What is the risk of cancer among steaming hot tea drinkers? The risk appears to be 0.68 or 68 per cent in the exposed group, and 0.2919 or 29 per cent in the unexposed group:

$$p_1 = \frac{a}{e} = \frac{65}{95} = 0.6842$$

Here is the calculation for the unexposed group:

$$p_0 = \frac{a}{f} = \frac{235}{805} = 0.2919$$

However, this is clearly not a sensible interpretation. Look at the overall risk of lung cancer (the prevalence of lung cancer) for this study:

$$p = \frac{g}{N} = \frac{300}{900} = 0.3333$$

It is 33 per cent, which is clearly far too high. A third of the population surely did not develop oesophageal cancer! In this study, researchers have deliberately chosen a set of controls, who do not have the disease, but are matched to patients who have the disease. This is a case-control study. They have selected twice as many controls as cases, but might have selected the same number, or more than twice as many. The number of cases to controls is not important. What is important is that the sample does not reflect the prevalence of the disease in the population. The risk of cancer is not 33 per cent, nor is it 68 per cent and 29 per cent in the exposed and unexposed groups. These people were selected artificially, to ensure that for each case, a control was selected who was as similar as possible to the case. We cannot calculate the risk of cancer here, because we do not know what the risk is for controls. The row and column totals are very misleading. We cannot calculate the risk, which means that we cannot calculate the relative risk either.

Table 4.7 Illustrative table showing numbers of people with risk (exposure) and disease (outcome)

	Disease present (cases)	*Disease absent (controls)*
Risk present	100	58
Risk absent	225	45

What we can do is calculate the relative odds, or odds ratio. It is meaningful to compare the odds of the disease among the exposed, to the odds of disease among the unexposed. Odds ratios were invented for case control studies for precisely this reason. Whereas relative risk concerns the ratio of events to the total number of events, odds ratios concern the ratio of events to non-events.

Having calculated odds ratios by hand, now try the same procedure using R for the following data. R will also provide a chi-square test of statistical significance and the associated *p*-value.

Box 4.2 R code for 2 × 2 tables (epibasix package)

The epibasix package was developed by Michael A Rotondi at the University of Western Ontario.

To install the epibasix packages, click on Packages, Install package(s) and then scroll down the list of packages to select epibasix.

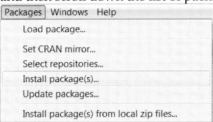

Figure 4.1 Installing a package in R

The command below creates a 2 × 2 table for analysis in the R epibasix package. Each column of values (100, 225) and (58, 45) is concatenated (joined together) using the cbind command. The summary command produces the chi-square statistic, *p* value, odds ratio, relative risk and risk difference. There are two different results for the risk difference, depending on whether the study was a cohort (Chapter 9) or case-control (Chapter 10) design.

```
require(epibasix) #this 'activates' the package, telling R
# that epibasix is required
data <- cbind(c(100, 225), c(58, 45)); #top to bottom, then
# left to right (a, c, b, d).

summary(epi2x2(data));
```

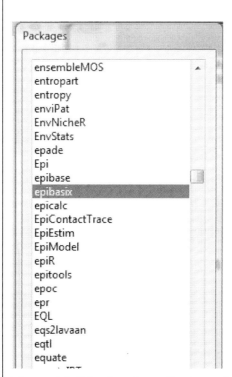

Figure 4.2 Selecting the epibasix package

```
> data <- cbind(c(100, 225), c(58, 45)); #top to bottom, then left to right (a, c, b, d).
> #A helpful way to remember this sequence is that the cell names have the same order in data<cbind
> summary(epi2x2(data));
Epidemiological 2x2 Table Analysis

Input Matrix:
            Disease Present (Cases) Disease Absent (Controls)
Risk Present            100                         58
Risk Absent             225                         45

Pearson Chi-Squared Statistic (Includes Yates' Continuity Correction): 20.827
Associated p.value for H0: There is an association between exposure and outcome vs. HA: No association : 0
p.value using Fisher's Exact Test (1 DF) : 0

Estimate of Odds Ratio: 0.345
95% Confidence Limits for true Odds Ratio are: [0.219, 0.544]

Estimate of Relative Risk (Cohort, Col1): 0.759
95% Confidence Limits for true Relative Risk are: [0.667, 0.865]

Estimate of Risk Difference (p1 - p2) in Cohort Studies: -0.2
95% Confidence Limits for Risk Difference: [-0.293, -0.108]

Estimate of Risk Difference (p1 - p2) in Case Control Studies: -0.255
95% Confidence Limits for Risk Difference: [-0.355, -0.156]

Note: Above Confidence Intervals employ a continuity correction.
```

Figure 4.3 Using the epibasix package

Box 4.3 Exercise: Calculating an odds ratio

This is the formula for calculating an odds ratio (OR), which you must use when data are from a case control study. We will use the study which investigated the odds of cancer for steaming hot tea drinkers, to illustrate. This study was a case control study, which means that we cannot calculate the relative risk. The odds ratio will approximate the relative risk.

$$OR = \frac{a/b}{c/d} = \frac{ad}{bc}$$

The equation rearranges to give ad/bc, but you can calculate a/b and c/d separately first, if you prefer. Calculating them separately will show you what the odds are in the exposed and unexposed groups. Either approach will ultimately provide the same answer. We will now try calculating the odds ratio for the hot tea study, and see if this provides a more meaningful interpretation.

$$OR = \frac{65/30}{235/570} = \frac{2.1667}{0.4123} = 5.26$$

Reporting at two decimal places, the odds ratio is 5.26. This suggests that there is a 5.26-fold increase in the odds of cancer in the exposed group, compared to the unexposed group. The interpretation is similar to that for risk ratio, but strictly speaking, they are not the same thing. We cannot really say that the odds are 5.26 times higher, but the odds ratio is usually a good approximation to the relative risk. The term 'fold' is used throughout this book, to help distinguish odds ratio ('five-fold increase') from a relative risk ('five times more likely'). This distinction is not always made in research reports, however, but should hopefully be clear from the context. Odds ratios can also be calculated for other study designs. If we calculate the odds ratio for lung cancer for smokers versus non-smokers, using the previous data, we obtain the following:

$$OR = \frac{39/29961}{6/59994} = \frac{0.0013}{0.0001} = 13$$

The odds ratio is 13, the same as the risk ratio of 13 we found previously for this data set. Odds ratios are similar to risk ratios, when the disease is rare. Table 4.8 shows how to calculate confidence intervals for odds ratios.

Table 4.8 Calculating CI for odds ratios

Maths notation	Example	In English
$SE \log OR = \sqrt{\dfrac{1}{a} + \dfrac{1}{b} + \dfrac{1}{c} + \dfrac{1}{d}}$	$SE \log OR = \sqrt{\dfrac{1}{100} + \dfrac{1}{58} + \dfrac{1}{225} + \dfrac{1}{45}}$ $= 0.2322$	Take the reciprocal of cells a, b, c and d. Add them together. Take the square root. This is the standard error of the log OR. Note that this equation is different from the equation for SElogRR, which involves different cells and different operators.
$EF = \exp\left(1.96 \left(SE \log OR\right)\right)$	$= \exp(1.96 \times 0.2322)$ $= 1.5764$	Multiply the standard error of the log OR by 1.96, then take the exponent of the result. This is the error factor.
$95\% CI = \dfrac{OR}{EF}, \quad OR \times EF$	$= 5.26 / 1.5764, \ 5.26 \times 1.5764$ $= 3.3367, 8.2919$	To obtain the lower confidence interval, divide the odds ratio by the error factor. For the upper interval, multiply the odds ratio by the error factor.
$z = \dfrac{\log OR}{SE \log OR}$	$= 1.6601 / 0.2322$ $= 7.15 \ (1 \ \text{d.f.})$	To obtain the z-statistic, divide the natural log of the odds ratio by the standard error of the log odds ratio. Looking up the z-value in the table in Appendix 2 shows that the probability of the data under the null hypothesis is very small ($p < .01$).

Summary: Drinking steaming hot tea was associated with oesophageal cancer (OR = 7.15, 95% CI 3.34 to 8.29, $p < .001$).

Why use odds ratios?

Initially, most students tend to prefer thinking about relative risks, than odds ratios, particularly early in their training. However, it is important to work with odds ratios as well. There are four reasons why we use odds ratios:

1 Risk ratios are not available in case control studies. Therefore, we have to rely on odds ratios to approximate the relative risk.

2 Odds ratios are used to adjust for confounding factors in multivariate models. That is, statistical models which take into account more than two variables. In real-life research, multivariate models are more typical and risk ratios are not available here.

3 Risk ratios become constrained for common events. That is, there is a 'ceiling effect' which makes the estimate unstable and less meaningful. In Table 4.9, you can clearly see that the odds ratio is 2 without even calculating it. However, the risk ratio is 1.33, which might surprise you. This is because the event is very common, constraining the risk ratio.

4 The interpretation of odds ratios is effectively the same as for risk ratios. Both refer to the relative occurrence or absence of an event of interest. Given that odds ratios address the first three points in the list, the sensible choice in most cases is to work with them.

Absolute versus relative risks

Suppose Lazar's disease, entirely fictional from the BBC's 'Doctor Who', is a rare disease. A drug representative arrives with some glossy promotional material, which claims that Hydromel reduces the risk of Lazar's disease by 80 per cent:

> Our drug reduces the risk of Lazar's disease by 80%!

> Start prescribing today!

They suggest that you start prescribing the drug. Intrigued, you contact the drug company and ask to see the raw data. They only provide the information in Table 4.9. Complete the table, and answer the following questions:

Table 4.9 Hypothetical data for Hydromel and Lazar's disease adapted from [25]

	Lazar's disease	Healthy	Total
Hydromel	1	9 999	
Unexposed	5	9 995	
Total			

1 Calculate the relative risk and interpret what it means.

2 Calculate the relative risk reduction (also known as the efficacy of the drug). Is the drug rep correct that the risk is reduced by 80 per cent?

3 Calculate the absolute risk difference. Would you be convinced enough to start prescribing Hydromel?

4 How many patients would have to be treated with Hydromel, to prevent one case of Lazar's disease?

5 Suppose that Hydromel would cost £1.60 per month per patient (5p per day). What is the cost of preventing one case of Lazar's?

Answers are available on the book website.

Box 4.4 An aside: Contraceptive use and risk of thrombosis

Is 'third generation' contraceptive use associated with increased risk of thrombosis? A meta-analysis published in the BMJ suggested that there is an association [28]. The odds ratio of 3.1 (95% confidence intervals 2.0 to 4.6; based on four studies) suggested a 3.1-fold increase in the risk of venous thromboembolism for women using third generation oral contraceptives rather than second generation oral contraceptives. The confidence intervals do not include 1, suggesting that the odds ratio is statistically significant. The odds ratio was adjusted for relevant confounding factors.

The absolute risk of thrombosis, for individuals using third generation contraceptives, presents a different picture. The authors report an excess risk of 1.5 per 10 000 woman years (for regular users) and 6.6 per 10 000 woman years (for new users). The excess risk corresponds to the absolute risk difference, which is just 0.00015 or 0.015 per cent. The risk to an individual is therefore extremely small indeed. It is only if we want to consider the relative risk (or odds ratio) across the whole population that this association becomes meaningful. Commentators noted that this increased risk should be balanced against the risk of thrombosis in pregnant women, reductions in unintended pregnancies and protective benefits offered by oral contraceptives against other kinds of morbidity and mortality [29].

Summary

Relative risks and odds ratios can mislead, because they provide no indication of the absolute risk to an individual associated with an exposure. The study in Box 4.4 is a good example of why it is essential to consider both absolute and relative risks. The appropriate way to communicate a risk depends on the intended audience, and this is particularly important when research findings are reported to the media. The public may not understand that a relative risk of 3.1, which the media might report as 'more than three times more likely' is consistent with an increase of 0.015 per cent in their own risk as a third generation contraceptive user. It is also worth noting that the odds ratio was different in studies conducted by the pharmaceutical industry (OR = 1.3, 95% CI 1.0 to 1.7) compared to other sources of funding (OR = 2.3, 95% CI 1.7 to 3.2). The consistency of an association across different studies is an important factor to consider when deciding if an association is causal or not (introduced later), and may be important when critically appraising a paper.

## 5

Measures of association for continuous outcomes

We often want to know whether an exposure or a treatment is associated with a continuous outcome variable. For example, is smoking associated with reduced walking speed? Does drug A lower blood pressure compared to drug B? Is negative emotionality associated with cholesterol? When the exposure is categorical, we want to know the difference between the two groups concerned on the outcome variable. How much slower do smokers walk than non-smokers? When the exposure is continuous, we want to know whether the exposure and outcome co-vary. For example do people with higher negative emotionality have higher cholesterol, meaning that they are positively correlated? Methods for determining the magnitude, confidence intervals and significance of such differences and relationships are introduced in this chapter. These methods build heavily on the standard error and confidence interval, which we learned about in the previous chapter.

Intended learning outcomes

By the end of this chapter, you should be able to:

- calculate the size of the difference between two groups exposed to a risk factor or a treatment;
- calculate confidence intervals around the estimated difference;
- determine whether this difference is statistically significant:
  - z- and T-test for differences in means
  - one-way ANOVA
  - z- and T-test for differences in means when data are paired (repeated measures)
  - non-parametric tests for ranked data
- calculate a correlation coefficient for two continuous variables;
- calculate confidence intervals around a correlation coefficient;
- determine if the correlation is statistically significant.

Differences between two means

In Chapter 1, we determined the magnitude, confidence and significance of the difference between a sample mean and a hypothesised value (the known population mean). In this chapter, we follow the same process, but consider the more common situation where two means from the sample are compared (or two means from the same people, measured at different times, in the same sample).

Assumptions of parametric tests

Some of the tests in this chapter are parametric tests, which require three assumptions to be met:

- the level of measurement for the dependent variable should be at least interval;

- normally distributed values in the population (although testing whether a distribution is normal can be controversial);

- similar variances (as a general rule, one no more than twice the size of the other [20]).

In practice, it is difficult to determine if data are normally distributed. There are tests available which compare the data to a normal distribution, but these tests can be too strict. Visually inspecting a histogram of the values is more typically done, but this can be too subjective, and it is difficult when working with small sample sizes. There is a plot called the Q-Q plot in R which can help, but this too involves subjective decision making. It is important to remember that the test assumes a normal distribution in the population, not the sample. Similarly, it is difficult to determine if variances are dissimilar enough to warrant concern, since many tests perform quite well even if the variances are different.

Box 5.1 R code for Q-Q plots

You can compare the data to how the data should look if they were normally distributed, using a Q-Q plot. The example below illustrates how to do this for the heights data.

```
data <- read.table('height.csv', header=TRUE, sep=',')
attach(data)
qqnorm(height, ylab = "Height (cm)", pch="+")
qqline(height)
points( qnorm(c(.25,.75)),quantile(height, c(.25, .75)) ,
pch=16, col=2, cex=2)
```

The data points (+) would lie on the solid line, if they were normally distributed. Although the data points in Figure 5.1 are tending towards normality, it appears that the distribution is non-normal. Given the small sample size (n=10) and the fact that we know height is normally distributed in the population, in this situation we can assume that the assumption of normality has been met.

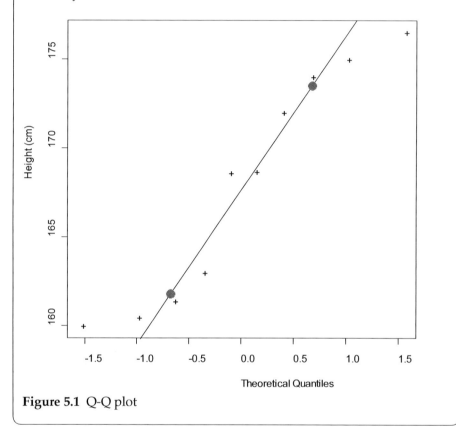

Figure 5.1 Q-Q plot

Z-test (large samples)

To perform the one-sample z-test, calculate the difference between the sample mean and the population mean, and divide it by the standard error of the difference:

$$z\frac{(x-\mu_0)}{(s/\sqrt{n})}$$

The z-test is suitable for large samples, and tests whether the observed mean in the sample is consistent with the hypothesized mean in the population.

Unrelated t-test (small samples)

The unrelated (Student's) *t*-test assumes that even if your data are not normally distributed, the population distribution from which they came is normal. It is preferable to the *z*-test when you have small samples, but when using a computer the results are unlikely to differ materially.

$$t = \frac{\bar{x}_1 - \bar{x}_2}{\text{SE}}, \qquad d.f. = n_1 + n_2 - 2$$

The *t*-statistic is calculated by subtracting the mean of the comparison group from the mean of the reference group, and dividing by their pooled standard error. This standard error of the difference between the two means should be calculated in the following way, and then you can insert this into the equation above:

$$\text{SE} = s \sqrt{\left(\frac{1}{n_1} + \frac{1}{n_0} \right)}$$

This is the standard deviation, multiplied by the square root of the sum of the inverse of each group's sample size. You first need, however, the common standard deviation:

$$s = \sqrt{\left[\frac{(n_1 - 1)s_1^2 + (n_0 - 1)s_0^2}{(n_1 + n_0 - 2)} \right]}$$

This is the pooled standard deviation, and although the formula looks complicated, you only need to calculate the standard deviation in each group, and the rest is relatively straightforward. When you have calculated the *t*-statistic, use the *t*-table in Appendix 1 and appropriate degrees of freedom to determine if the two groups have significantly different means or not. In the unrelated *t*-test, the degrees of freedom are always the total sample size minus two, the number of groups. A complete example is shown below.

Worked example

Waist–hip ratio (WHR) is calculated by dividing waist size (cm) by girth at the hips (cm), usually the widest point or the mean of several measurements. WHR is used variously as an indicator of adiposity, physical fitness and health status. Empirical support for these claims is provided by evidence that higher waist–hip ratios are associated with all-cause mortality risk, and cardiovascular mortality risk in particular. Our interest however, for this exercise, is simply to test whether a sample of men and women actually have different WHRs. Using a small data set, we will test the hypothesis that men have higher WHRs. This is a one-tailed hypothesis, because we have made a prediction about the direction of the difference (males = higher).

The *t*-statistic obtained is 2.34, which is greater than the cut point of 2.10 for a two-tailed test at $p < .05$. Therefore, we reject the null hypothesis that any

Table 5.1 Data for waist–hip ratio

	WHR (males, group 1)	$x - \bar{x}$	$(x - \bar{x})^2$	WHR (females, group 0)	$x - \bar{x}$	$(x - \bar{x})^2$
1	0.91	0.00	0.00	0.84	0.00	0.00
2	0.98	0.07	0.01	0.79	−0.05	0.00
3	0.90	−0.01	0.00	0.98	0.14	0.02
4	0.89	−0.02	0.00	0.73	−0.11	0.01
5	0.86	−0.05	0.00	0.76	−0.08	0.01
6	0.94	0.03	0.00	0.85	0.01	0.00
7	0.86	−0.05	0.00	0.94	0.10	0.01
8	0.83	−0.08	0.01	0.85	0.01	0.00
9	0.98	0.07	0.01	0.84	0.00	0.00
10	0.92	0.01	0.00	0.82	−0.02	0.00
Total	9.07		0.02	8.40		0.05
N	10			10		
Mean	0.91			0.84		
SD	0.0501			0.0754		

Difference between means

$$0.91 - 0.84 = 0.067$$

Common SD

$$s = \sqrt{\left[\frac{(n_1 - 1)s_1^2 + (n_0 - 1)s_0^2}{(n_1 + n_0 - 2)} \right]}$$

$$s = \sqrt{\left[\frac{(10 - 1)(0.0501^2) + (10 - 1)(0.0754^2)}{(10 + 10 - 2)} \right]}$$

$$s = \sqrt{\left[\frac{0.07381}{18} \right]} = 0.0640$$

SE of difference between means

$$SE = s\sqrt{\left(\frac{1}{n_1} + \frac{1}{n_0} \right)}$$

$$SE = 0.0640\sqrt{\left(\frac{1}{10} + \frac{1}{10} \right)} = 0.0286$$

T statistic

$$t = \frac{\bar{x}_1 - \bar{x}_2}{se} = \frac{0.91 - 0.84}{0.0286} = 2.34$$

Degrees of freedom

$$d.f. = n_1 + n_2 - 2 = 10 + 10 - 2 = 18$$

$p < .05$ (see t-table in Appendix 1)

Exact p value

This was obtained from Excel.

$p = .02$

difference between the means is due to chance. The probability of our data, if the null hypothesis were true, is very small (less than 5 per cent, as indicated by a p value less than .05). The exact p value can be obtained in Excel, R or other statistical software. As with all statistics, it is important to calculate confidence intervals in addition to determining the magnitude and significance of the differences observed. The method for calculating confidence intervals for an unrelated t-test is shown below.

Confidence intervals

In the formulae below, you need to replace t with the appropriate value from the t-distribution (Appendix 1). This depends on the percentage point, and the (two-sided) degrees of freedom. For 18 degrees of freedom, the correct value is 2.10. If the sample sizes are different from 10 in each group, this value should be changed as required.

$$\text{lowerCI} = (\bar{x}_1 - \bar{x}_0) - (t \times \text{SE}) = (0.0670) - (2.10 \times 0.0286) = 0.01$$

$$\text{upperCI} = (\bar{x}_1 - \bar{x}_0) + (t \times se) = (0.0670) + (2.10 \times 0.0286) = 0.13$$

The results suggest that men have a significantly higher WHR than women, consistent with [20] a small difference to a moderate difference ($t = 2.34$, mean difference = 0.07, 95% CI 0.01 to 0.13, $p < .05$). This is a concise way of summarising what we have found, and is typically what to expect in a journal article. Most academic journals in the health sciences will now insist that the exact p value is reported, rather than the historic tradition of reporting either $p < .05$ (significant) or $p < .01$ (highly significant). Some epidemiology journals do not allow p values at all, preferring to report confidence intervals only. We return to these issues in the critical appraisal chapters.

Box 5.2 R code for unrelated t-test

This method produces equivalent results to the example shown by hand, and to the t.test function available in R. It uses however, the regression method (Chapter 13) which treats the t-test as a special case of multiple regression, where there is only one categorical predictor (sex). Sex is coded 1 for male and 2 for female.

```
data <- read.table('whr.csv',
header=TRUE, sep=',')
attach(data)
library(gplots)
sex<- factor(sex)
plotmeans(whr~sex,xlab="Sex",ylab="WHR", main="Mean Plot\n
with 95% CI") #\n creates a line break
male <- (sex=="1")*1 #dummy variable for male
female <- (sex=="2")*1 #dummy variable for female
```

```
results<- lm(whr~male)  #produces the same t value as by hand
summary(results)
```

The graph in Figure 5.2 shows that the mean WHR for males is higher than the mean WHR for females, and also that there is more variance among females. The regression line connecting the two group means is a significantly better fit to the data than is relying on the overall mean (0.8735). We return to regression lines in more detail in Chapter 13.

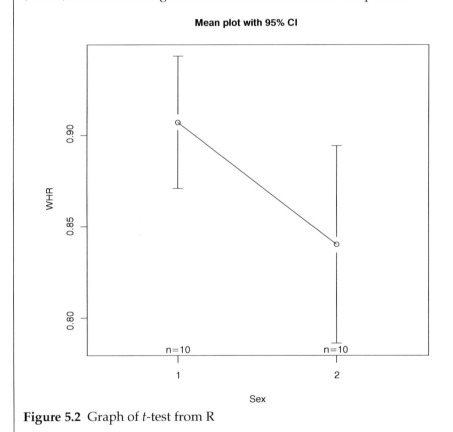

Figure 5.2 Graph of *t*-test from R

t-test for repeated measures (paired) data

It often happens that data are paired, so that the observations are not independent. For example, scores on a test could be measured before and after some intervention, on the same people. In case-control studies, two different people are measured on the same variable, but their scores are not independent – the data are paired. When data are paired, it is not appropriate to conduct a *t*- or *z*-test on their difference in means. Instead, use one of the following formulae, depending on the sample size:

$$z = \frac{\overline{x}}{\text{SE}} = \frac{\overline{x}}{s/\sqrt{n}}$$

$$t = \frac{\overline{x}}{\text{SE}} = \frac{\overline{x}}{s/\sqrt{n'}} \qquad d.f. = 1$$

To illustrate with an example, suppose that General Health Questionnaire (GHQ-12) score was measured using a computerised test, and a paper and pencil version (counterbalanced, so that a random half of participants received the computerised version first). The hypothesis is that there would be no significant difference between the two conditions, supporting the use of either version.

The formula for calculating a 95 per cent confidence interval around the mean differences is slightly different than before, because we have ten pairs, meaning nine degrees of freedom are available. The five per cent point is 2.26 in the t table, when there are nine degrees of freedom.

$$\text{CI} = \overline{x} \pm (z \times \text{SE}) \quad (>=60 \text{ pairs})$$

$$\text{CI} = \overline{x} \pm (t \times \text{SE}) \quad (<60 \text{ pairs})$$

Table 5.2 *t*-test for repeated measures (paired) data

ID	Paper condition	Computer condition	Difference
1	18	8	10.0000
2	19	18	1.0000
3	17	22	−5.0000
4	13	20	−7.0000
5	18	11	7.0000
6	18	18	0.0000
7	12	17	−5.0000
8	20	17	3.0000
9	15	12	3.0000
10	20	26	-6.0000
Mean		Mean difference	0.1
		Variance	33.6667
		SD of differences	5.8023
		SE of mean	1.8348
		t	0.0545
		d.f.	9
	See text for calculation	Lower interval	−4.0500
	See text for calculation	Upper interval	4.2500
		p	0.96

We have a small sample of nine pairs. The standard error of the differences is 1.8348, therefore:

0.1– (2.26 × 1.8348) = –4.046648

0.1+ (2.26 × 1.8348) = 4.246648

The results show that there is only a very small difference between GHQ-12 scores in each condition (0.1 points, 95% CI). The probability that we observe this result, if the null hypothesis of no difference were true, is very high (p = 0.96). The confidence intervals include zero, also suggesting no significant or reliable difference between the scores in each condition (mean difference = 0.1, 95% CI –4.05 to 4.24).

One-way ANOVA

One-way analysis of variance (ANOVA) is used to test the differences between means in more than two groups. The unrelated t-test should not be used when there are three or more groups. For example, which of three dietary interventions lead to the lowest systolic blood pressure at follow-up six months later (Table 5.3)? In this hypothetical data, 30 participants have been randomly assigned to three groups, each given a different dietary intervention. Here, we cannot use the independent t-test to compare three groups at the same time.

ANOVA partitions the variance in the dependent variable (total variability) into two parts: the variability between the groups (between-groups variance) and variability within the groups (within-groups variance). The variability between the groups is most important to us, because that concerns the effect of each diet on the outcome (blood pressure). Variation within the groups is not due to diet, this reflects individual differences and other random error. Assuming that participants have been randomly assigned to each diet, we can therefore consider variation within groups to be ramdon error for our purposes. If the diets had no effect on systolic blood pressure, the variability between

Table 5.3 Data for three-group dietary intervention

Diet A	Diet B	Diet C
129	131	107
135	127	106
141	151	122
108	120	141
119	129	141
146	113	157
112	154	133
161	176	114
122	117	119
129	126	118

Table 5.4 Total variation

Maths notation	Example	Result	In English
$\sum x$	$1302+1344+1258$	3904	Add up all the x values (Table 5.3) in the data set (column A total + column B total + column C total)
$\sum x^2$	$[16641+18225+19881+11664+14161+21316+12544+25921+14884+16641]$ $+[17161+16129+22801+14400+16641+12769+23716+30976+13689+15876]$ $+[11449+11236+14884+19881+24649+17689+12996+14161+13924]$	516786	Add up the squared x values in each column (columns are shown in squared brackets but these are not needed in the calculation – add them all together)
$\sum (x-\bar{x})^2$ $=\sum x^2 - (\sum x)^2 / n$	$516786 - 39042/30$	8745.4667	Subtract the total from the squared total, then divide by the sample size
Degrees of freedom	30-1	29	Subtract 1 from the sample size

Table 5.5 Between groups variation

Maths notation	Example	Result	In English
$\sum n_i \bar{x}_i^2 - (\sum x)^2 / n$	$10 \times 130.22 + 10 \times 134.42 \times 125.82/30$	369.8667	Multiply the sample size by the mean squared in each group, add them together, divide by the sample size
Degrees of freedom	$k - 1 = 3 - 1$	2	Subtract 1 from the number of groups

Table 5.6 Within groups variation

Maths notation	Example	Result	In English
$\sum (n_i - 1)s_i^2$	$10 - 1 \times 16.185\ 10 - 1 \times 19.7889$ $+ 10 - 1 \times 16.6453$	8375.6	Multiply the squared standard deviation in each group by the sample size in each group minus 1, add together.
Degrees of freedom	$n - k = 30-3$	27	Subtract the number of groups from the sample size

groups would be the same as the variability within groups. Therefore, the ratio of between-group variance to within-group variance would be 1. This is the variance ratio test, which produces the F-statistic. If the F-statistic is significantly different from 1, then the means are significantly different, suggesting that diet did have an effect on systolic blood pressure.

There are five steps to performing a one-way ANOVA by hand, outlined below:

1. check that the variances in each group are not substantially different;

2. calculate the total variation;

3. calculate the between-groups variation;

4. calculate the within-groups variation;

5. calculate the F-statistic, which is the ratio of between- to within-group variance $F = \dfrac{s_1^2}{s_0^2}$. Here 1 is the larger variance and 0 is the smaller variance [30].

This gives

$$F = \frac{s_1^2}{s_0^2} = \frac{391.6}{261.9556} = 1.5$$

The largest variance is not twice as large as the smallest, suggesting that the variances are not significantly different. To calculate the degrees of freedom, subtract 1 from n (group 1) and m (group 2). We have ten people in each group so there are 9 and 9 degrees of freedom. In Appendix 2, the critical value can be found by selecting the appropriate row (9) and column (9) for these particular degrees of freedom. Our result of 1.5 does not exceed the critical value of 3.18, showing that the variances are indeed not significantly different. This satisfies the assumption of equality of variances, and we can therefore proceed with the ANOVA. The calculations and explanations are given in Tables 5.4 to 5.7

Having obtained the F-statistic, we can now look at the F table (Appendix 2) and find out if our F value of 0.60 exceeds the critical value shown, with 2 (row) and 27 (column) degrees of freedom. The nearest critical value is 3.316, and therefore we have not found evidence that the means are significantly different. The three diets resulted in similar systolic blood pressure values at follow-up.

One limitation of ANOVA is that when significant differences are found between groups, it is not immediately clear which group this might refer

Table 5.7 Variance ratio: table of result

In English	Value	Degrees of freedom	Mean square	F statistic
Maths notation		df		
Between groups	369.8667	2	184.9333	0.60
Within groups	8375.6	27	310.2074	
Total	8745.4667	29		

Box 5.3 R code for one-way ANOVA

The ANOVA function in R produces different results to the method in this chapter, because it uses a different method for calculating sum of squares. The reasons for this are not crucially important at an introductory level, but you can read more about this issue elsewhere [31]. To obtain comparable results in R, it is better to run ANOVA as a regression model. ANOVA is a special case of regression (introduced in Chapter 13) in which a single predictor variable is a categorical variable (here, type of diet) rather than a continuous variable. The results are exactly the same, whether calculating the F-statistic using ANOVA or regression. The regression line is the line of best fit, when connecting the three means together. As shown in the plot below, there is a steady decrease in mean systolic blood pressure as we compare diet 1, diet 2 and diet 3. The question is, whether these differences are significantly different, or due to chance. We should also ask whether the differences are clinically significant, which is discussed in Chapter 12. Focusing on whether the differences are statistically significant, another way of phrasing the question is to consider whether the regression line is a better model of the data than simply using the grand mean. If the mean systolic blood pressure for all groups describes the data well, then why bother attempting to model the differences in means across groups?

If the regression line is steep enough, this would imply that there is more variation between the groups than variation within the groups. In our example, we can see that there is more variation within the groups, than between them. The confidence intervals overlap each other, which is a useful way to visually determine if group differences are significant. The F-ratio test confirms that there is a high probability that the differences observed are consistent with the null hypothesis.

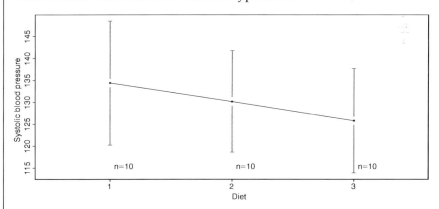

```
data <- read.table('diets.csv', header=TRUE, sep=',')
attach(data)
names(data)
#Visual results, adapted from http://www.statmethods.net/
# stats/anova.html
```

```
library(gplots)
diet <- factor(diet)
plotmeans(sbp~diet,xlab="Diet",ylab="Systolic blood
pressure", main="Mean Plot\n with 95% CI") #\n creates a
# line break
d1 <- (diet=="1")*1 #dummy variable for diet 1
d2 <- (diet=="2")*1 #dummy variable for diet 2
d3 <- (diet=="3")*1 #dummy variable for diet 3
results<- lm(sbp~d1+d3) #produces the same F value as ANOVA
```

Chapter 13 will explain how to interpret the results from the regression output. For now, the important thing to note is that the F-value is the same as that calculated by hand.

to. Methods do exist that allow us to find out where the differences lie. A straightforward method for doing this is shown in chapter 13, on regression models.

Continuous exposure (correlation, covariance)

The association between two continuous variables (e.g. strength and speed) can be measured by their covariance and by their correlation coefficient (example Table 5.8 from [32]). Covariance and correlation are similar, but the correlation coefficient is standardised to range from –1 to 1 .

$$r = \frac{\sum (x - \bar{x})(y - \bar{y})}{\sqrt{\left[\sum (x - \bar{x})^2 \sum (y - \bar{y})^2\right]}}$$

Ranked data

Wilcoxon rank sum test [Mann-Whitney U test] (for unpaired data)

The data in Table 5.9 are from a real data set, a nice example included within the R program. They are permeability constants for chorioamnion values, a placental membrane, at term and at 12–26 weeks gestational age. Chorioamnion is hypothesised to be more permeable for pregnancies at term.

In this test, we first rank the data together in ascending (lowest to highest) order, giving the same rank to any values that are the same. Make sure you rank both groups together. Ignore any missing values, for example, if the sample sizes are different. Next, take the sum of the ranks in each group. Here, they are 90 and 30. The sum of the ranks in the smaller group ($N = 5$) provides the T-statistic (not to be confused with the t-test), sometimes called the U-statistic. In Appendix 4, if our T/U is smaller than the value shown in the table, we

Table 5.8 Calculation of correlation coefficient

x	y	x-mean	y-mean	Cross products	x-mean^2	y-mean^2
21.6	135	−1.94	−38.00	73.72	3.76	1444.00
23.4	213	−0.14	40.00	−5.60	0.02	1600.00
26.5	243	2.96	70.00	207.20	8.76	4900.00
25.5	167	1.96	−6.00	−11.76	3.84	36.00
20.8	120	−2.74	−53.00	145.22	7.51	2809.00
19.5	134	−4.04	−39.00	157.56	16.32	1521.00
20.9	209	−2.64	36.00	−95.04	6.97	1296.00
18.7	176	−4.84	3.00	−14.52	23.43	9.00
29.8	156	6.26	−17.00	−106.42	39.19	289.00
28.7	177	5.16	4.00	20.64	26.63	16.00
Mean = 23.54	Mean = 173.00	A: Sum of cross products		371.00	136.42	13920.00

B: product of sum of squared deviations from the mean: 136.42 × 13920 = 1899022.08

C: Square root of B   1378.05

D: Correlation coefficient (A/C): $r = 0.27$

R code   `cor(x,y)#where x and y are two continuous variables`

Table 5.9 Data for permeability constants for chorioamnion values

Chorioamnion at term	Rank	Chorioamnion at 12–26 weeks	Rank
0.8	1	1.15	1
0.83	3	0.88	3
1.89	4	0.9	4
1.04	7	0.74	7
1.45	10	1.21	10
1.38	11	NA	
1.91	12	NA	
1.64	13	NA	
0.73	14	NA	
1.46	15	NA	
Sum of ranks	90	Sum of ranks	30

T = sum of ranks in group with smaller $N = 30$

W = sum of ranks in larger group – sum of ranks in smaller group = 90 – 30 = 60

> **Box 5.4** R code for Mann Whitney U test
>
> ```
> data <- read.table('chorioamnion.csv', header=TRUE, sep=',',
> na.strings="NA")
> attach(data)
> names(data)
> wilcox.test(x,y,paired=FALSE,correct=FALSE) #note that R
> # produces the W not the T statistic
> ```

reject the null hypothesis. Our value of 30 is larger than the critical value of 8 (for $N = 5$ and $N = 10$), suggesting a high probability that this difference is due to chance. Note that our hypothesis is one-tailed, because we did have a specific direction for our hypothesis.

Wilcoxon signed rank test (for paired data)

Suppose a researcher wanted to determine whether a standard leaflet about breast cancer screening, or an interactive game designed to highlight risk factors for breast cancer, were better at increasing awareness of these risk factors. The design was a repeated measures design, counterbalanced so that a random half of participants read the leaflet first, and a random half did the game first. All women took part in both conditions, producing paired data. Scores were the number of correctly identified risk factors, ranging from 0 to 7. The data however, are considered nonparametric because the differences are not normally distributed. The median score is 5 for the leaflet and 7

Table 5.10 Wilcoxon signed rank test

	Leaflet	Game	Difference	Rank	Positive	Negative
1	6	6	0	NA		
2	7	7	0	NA		
3	7	7	0	NA		
4	4	7	–3	3.5		3.5
5	7	7	0	NA		
6	4	7	–3	3.5		3.5
7	7	3	4	6	6	
8	3	6	–3	3.5		3.5
9	2	3	–1	1		1
10	4	7	–3	3.5		3.5
Median	5	7		Sum + ranks	6	
				Sum – ranks	15	
				T	6	(smaller)
				N	6	

for the game, indicating that women are better at correctly identifying risk factors after the game. To determine if this is significantly different however, a nonparametric equivalent to the related *t*-test is required.

The Wilcoxon signed rank test begins by calculating the difference between the scores in the game and the leaflet conditions. Any zero differences are ignored. Next, the differences scores are assigned a rank from smallest to largest, ignoring the sign. Any tied ranks, ranks that have the same value, are averaged and assigned the same rank score. The difference score of –1 is given the rank 1. There are four scores with the value of 3 which are given the rank 3.5, because they occupy positions 2, 3, 4 and 5:

$$(2 + 3 + 4 + 5) / 4 = 3.5$$

The score of 4 is given rank 6. Because the four zero differences are ignored, our sample size is actually 6 rather than 10.

The next step is to add up the positive and negative ranks separately. The sum of positive ranks is 6, and the sum of negative ranks is 15. The *T*-statistic, which is not to be confused with the *t*-test, is the smaller of these two values. If the null hypothesis were true, the two values would be similar. If the null hypothesis is false, and there is a difference, then one will be smaller and one will be larger. The smaller value is used for the Wilcoxon test and is compared to the values in Wilcoxon table (Appendix 5). The differences are significant if our *T* is less than the value shown in the table (the critical value). Our sample size (*N*) is 6, because we ignored four zero differences. For a one-sided test and *p* at 0.05, the critical value shown in the table is 2. Our value of *T* is 6, which is greater than 2. Therefore, the differences are consistent with the null hypothesis. This could be a chance finding. The sample size however, was quite small, and we may not have enough statistical power to detect a reliable difference (see Appendix 7: Statistical Power).

Box 5.5 R code for Wilcoxon signed ranks test

```
data <- read.table('leaflet-game.csv', header=TRUE, sep=',')
attach(data)
names(data)
wilcox.test(game, leaflet, paired = TRUE, alternative =
"greater") #The V statistic is the same as T
```

Spearman's rho (correlation for nonparametric data)

The data in Table 5.11 are taken from a Health and Lifestyle Survey in Wakefield in 2008 [33], which included measures of alcohol use at the last sexual encounter (event-level sexual behaviour) and of mental health. Mental health was measured using the General Health Questionnaire 12 (GHQ-12). The number of drinks at the last sexual encounter is nonparametric, since several people drank nothing at all and some people reported many drinks. The data are not normally distributed. Additionally, it is questionable whether

Table 5.11 Spearman's rho

Number of drinks prior to last sexual event	Rank	GHQ-12 score	Rank
0	2	18	3.5
0	2	24	7
0	2	24	7
1	4	15	2
2	5	12	1
3	6	27	10
4	7	18	3.5
9	8	24	7
15	9	25	9
20	10	19	5

number of drinks is interval data, even if it were normally distributed. For these reasons, a Pearson correlation coefficient is not appropriate. Spearman's rho is a nonparametric version, which assigns ranks to the data rather than using the actual values. It is fairly straightforward to calculate. First we rank the data for each variable separately, then simply calculate the Pearson correlation coefficient on the ranks, not the data.

Summary

This chapter has introduced methods for identifying associations between continuous outcome variables. For example, we used a *t*-test to identify differences in means. We calculated correlation coefficients to summarise how strongly two continuous variables are associated with each other, and we used methods for ranked (ordinal) data. We also calculated confidence intervals for these statistics, as we did for measures of association for categorical outcomes in the previous chapter.

## 6

Confounding, effect modification, mediation and causal inference

Intended learning outcomes

By the end of this chapter, you should be able to:

- distinguish between confounding, effect modification, mediation and antecedent variables;
- adjust an odds ratio to control for confounding in a simple 2 × 2 table;
- summarise odds ratios for different levels of an effect modifier;
- evaluate the criteria for determining if an association is causal;
- situations in which a variable or mechanism may mediate or transmit the effect of an exposure on an outcome variable.

Introducing key terms

In previous chapters we have mostly been concerned with simple situations in which an exposure (X) is associated with a health outcome (Y). In reality, determining whether X has caused Y is rarely this simple [34]. There are at least five ways in which X and Y might *appear* to be related, and each may require different models or ways of thinking about the data:

1 confounding variables

2 effect modifying variables

3 mediating variables

4 antecedent variables

5 causal variables

It is important to become familiar with these different scenarios, particularly when critically appraising research articles. Few researchers are able to evaluate all of the possible scenarios that might have generated their data, particularly within the same paper or often within the same study. This chapter will introduce the five scenarios, provide an example of each, and suggest an appropriate method for estimating the association between X and Y in each. The first four scenarios concern a third variable A.

Confounding variables

Confounding occurs when the third variable A is associated both with X and with Y. Ignoring the confounding role of A would lead to a distorted estimate of the association between X and Y. The term 'confound' originates from Latin, where it meant to confuse or to puzzle. Confounding can indeed produce confusing or puzzling results. Consider, for example, a study which claims to have found an association between heavy alcohol drinking (X) and lung cancer (Y). The researchers find an odds ratio of 1.5 for heavy (vs. moderate) alcohol drinking and subsequent lung cancer. Would you believe that this association is genuine? Probably not, because we know from several decades of prior research that heavy alcohol drinkers are more likely to smoke. Is it more likely that smoking is causing the apparent association between alcohol and lung cancer? Because there tend to be more smokers among heavy alcohol drinkers, this creates a spurious or confounded association. Smoking is said to be a confounding factor because it is causally related to X and Y. A second example is the apparent association between keeping pet birds and lung cancer [35–39]. Smoking is a confounding variable in this example, because people who keep pet birds are more likely to smoke, and smoking is associated with lung cancer. In both examples, the arrows point from A to both X and Y which is an important criterion for determining whether confounding is plausible.

Confounding can distort results in different ways:

- producing an apparent association between X and Y where none exists;
- creating a larger association between X and Y than the smaller one which actually exists;
- creating a smaller association between X and Y than the larger one which actually exists.

What we want to find out is the true association between X and Y, once confounding factors have been considered. This could be no association

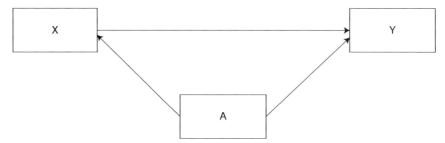

Figure 6.1 Confounding variables

(OR = 1), a negative association (OR < 1) or a positive association (OR > 1). Until we take the confounder (*A*) into account, often we do not know how much distortion has taken place. This is normally addressed by adjusting (controlling, or 'holding constant') the association for *A* in regression models, which we will consider in Chapters 13 and 14. Below, we will use a simplified method for summarising the adjusted OR in a simple 2 × 2 table. It is useful to calculate this by hand at least once, in order to familiarise yourself with how confounding works.

Addressing confounding in a simple 2 × 2 table

The Mantel–Haenszel odds ratio (OR) is an adjusted OR, taking into account the confounding factor A. First we calculate the OR separately in each stratum. Next, we calculate weights to determine how much each stratum should contribute to the summary OR. Finally, we calculate the summary OR, which is weighted to allow for the fact that the sample sizes differ in different strata.

$$OR = \frac{ad}{bc}$$

$$weight = \frac{cb}{n}$$

Do these two separately in each stratum, so that you have OR_1 and $weight_1$ for the first stratum, and OR_2 and $weight_2$ for the second stratum. Finally, combine the values to produce the Mantel–Haenszel OR.

$$OR_{MH} = \frac{(weight_1 OR_1) + (weight_2 OR_2)}{weight_1 + weight_2}$$

Here is an example; data are again from a study in Wakefield about alcohol and sexual health [33]. Participants completed a questionnaire that included questions on unprotected sexual intercourse in the last six months, and the Alcohol Use Disorders Identification Test (AUDIT) where scores of 8 or more were classified as hazardous drinking patterns. Our research question concerns whether hazardous alcohol drinking patterns (the exposure) are associated with unprotected sexual intercourse (the outcome). Having one or more unprotected penetrative sexual partner (PSP) is classified as the outcome. We also want to consider the potentially confounding role of gender, which could be associated both with the exposure and the outcome.

Table 6.1 shows the 2 × 2 tables for women and men separately, and the combined table. Calculating the overall OR on the combined table might produce an estimate of the OR which is confounded by sex. We want to calculate the Mantel–Haenszel OR.

In both men and women, a hazardous alcohol drinking pattern is associated with 1+ PSPs (OR = 1.34), although the estimate is a little larger for men (OR = 1.88). The combined estimate is OR = 1.49 which indicates a nearly 50 per cent increase in risk, adjusting for sex. This adjusted OR lies between the OR for men and women, as we might expect. Had we ignored the confounding role of sex,

Table 6.1 Calculating Mantel–Haenszel odds ratio

	Women			Men			Total		
	1+ PSP in last six months	0 PSP	Total	1+ PSP in last six months	0 PSP	Total	1+ PSP in last six months	0 PSP	Total
Hazardous drinking pattern	42	12	54	23	10	33	65	22	87
Non-hazardous drinking pattern	60	23	86	11	9	20	71	32	103
Total	102	35	137	34	19	53	136	54	190

$OR_{women} = ad/bc$
$OR_{women} = (42 \times 23) / (12 \times 60) = 1.34$
$weight_{women} = cb/n$
$weight_{women} = 60 \times 12 / 137 = 5.26$

$OR_{men} = ad/bc$
$OR_{men} = (23 \times 9) / (10 \times 11) = 1.88$
$weight_{men} = cb/n$
$weight_{men} = 11 \times 10 / 53 = 2.08$

$OR_{unadjusted} = ad/bc$
$OR_{unadjusted} =(65 \times 32) / (22 \times 71)$
$OR_{unadjusted} = 1.3$

$OR_{MH} = [(weight_{women} \times OR_{women}) + (weight_{men} \times OR_{men})] / (weigh_{twomen} + weight_{men})$
$OR_{MH} =[(5.26 \times 1.34) + (2.08 \times 1.88)] / (5.26 + 2.08)$
$OR_{MH} =1.49$

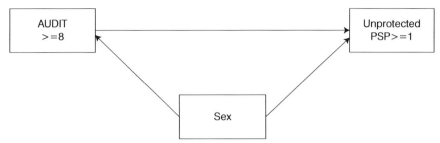

Figure 6.2 Confounding variable in the alcohol and sexual health study

we might have falsely concluded that the OR was 1.33. The estimate of 1.33 is not adjusted for sex, and is sometimes called a 'crude' estimate of the OR. It is likely to be biased. The true OR is likely to be around 1.49, higher than we would have estimated before calculating the adjusted OR. In this example, the adjusted OR is not statistically significant which could reflect low power because the sample size is small. It is consistent however, with an increase in risk.

Confidence interval for the adjusted OR

The formula for calculating a confidence interval for the adjusted OR (OR_{MH}) is [20]:

$$\frac{OR_{MH}}{EF} \qquad to \qquad OR_{MH}EF$$

We first need to calculate the error factor (EF). This can be worked out in a series of steps, each involving separate formulae, ending with the error factor calculation (note that Q, R and V are arbitrary values used to represent three different steps).

1 calculate Q

2 calculate R

3 calculate V

4 calculate the standard error of the adjusted OR, SE_{MH}

5 calculate the error factor (EF)

6 calculate the OR_{MH}, using a quick method

7 calculate the lower confidence interval

8 calculate the upper confidence interval

We will now work through these sequentially using the data above. In the equations that follow, the notation has been intentionally simplified. Several of the formulas below involve calculations being performed on each stratum (for men, for women) separately and then added together. When using full notation, subscripts are used to indicate that calculations should be done on each stratum separately. The sigma symbol (Σ) is used to indicate that these results should be added together. To reduce visual clutter, we will use a simplified version of the notation which does not show the subscript as in the table below:

Example of simplified notation used in this book	What this means (using full notation)	What you should do
$Q = \sum \dfrac{ad}{n}$	$Q = \sum \dfrac{a_i d_i}{n_i}$	$Q = \left(\dfrac{a_{men} d_{men}}{n_{men}} \right) + \left(\dfrac{a_{women} d_{women}}{n_{women}} \right)$

As usual, we will work at four significant figures and round to two significant figures at the last step.

- Step 1. Calculate **Q**

Maths notation	Example	Result	In English
$Q = \sum \dfrac{ad}{n}$	$Q_{men} = \dfrac{23 \times 9}{53}$ $= 3.9057$ $Q_{women} = \dfrac{42 \times 23}{137}$ $= 7.0511$	10.9568	Multiply a by d and divide by n. Do this separately for men and women. Add the answers together.

- Step 2. Calculate **R**

Maths notation	Example	Result	In English
$R = \sum \dfrac{cb}{n}$	$R_{men} = \dfrac{11 \times 10}{53}$ $= 2.0755$ $R_{women} = \dfrac{60 \times 12}{137}$ $= 5.2555$	7.3310	Multiply c by b and divide by n. Do this separately for men and women. Add the answers together.

- Step 3. Calculate **V**

V stands for 'variance' and captures the variability across the strata.

Maths notation	Example	Result	In English
$V = \sum \dfrac{ghef}{n^2(n-1)}$	$V_{men} = \dfrac{34 \times 19 \times 33 \times 20}{53^2(53-1)}$ $= 2.918914$ $V_{women} = \dfrac{102 \times 35 \times 54 \times 86}{137^2(137-1)}$ $= 6.495018$	9.4139	(1) Multiply g, h, e and f. (2) Divide by n-squared multiplied by $n{-}1$. Divide (1) by (2) Do this separately for men and women and add the answers together.

- Step 4. Calculate the standard error of the adjusted OR, SE_{MH}.

Maths notation	Example	Resault	In English
$SE_{MH} = \sqrt{\left[\dfrac{V}{QR}\right]}$	$SE_{MH} = \sqrt{\left[\dfrac{9.4139}{10.9568 \times 7.3309}\right]}$	0.3424	Divide V by $Q \times R$. Take the square root.

- Step 5. Calculate the error factor, EF.

In Maths	Example	Result	In English
$EF = \exp(1.96 \times SE_{MH})$	$EF = \exp(1.96 \times 0.3423)$ $EF = \exp(0.6710)$	1.9562	Multiply the standard error by 1.96. Take the exponent.

- Step 6. Calculate the OR_{MH}, using a quick method.

This step allows you to calculate the adjusted OR using a quick method, dividing Q by R. It gives nearly the same result (1.50) due to rounding error, and so is equivalent to the calculations we did above.

Maths notation	Example	Result	In English
$OR_{MH} = \dfrac{Q}{R}$	$OR_{MH} = \dfrac{10.9568}{7.3309}$	1.4946	Divide Q by R.

- Step 7. Calculate the lower confidence interval.

Maths notation	Example	Result	In English
Lower interval: $\dfrac{OR_{MH}}{EF}$	$\dfrac{1.4946}{1.9562}$	0.7640	Divide the adjusted (MH) odds ratio by the error factor.

- Step 8. Calculate the upper confidence interval.

Maths notation	Example	Result	In English
Upper interval: $OR_{MH} \times EF$	1.4946×1.9562	2.9237	Multiply the adjusted (MH) odds ratio by the error factor

In summary, the adjusted odds ratio is 1.49 (95% CI 0.76 to 2.92). This means that on this occasion, the adjusted odds ratio is not statistically significant (the confidence intervals include 1).

Effect modifying variables

In the second scenario, A could modify the association between X and Y. This means that the association is different, depending on the level of A. Effect modification is also called 'interaction' (particularly in psychology and other behavioural sciences), or 'heterogeneity between strata'. All of the following situations are hypothetical examples of effect modification:

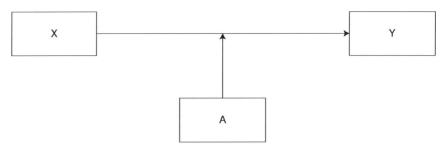

Figure 6.3 Effect modifying variables

- X has a stronger effect on Y in men than in women;
- X has a stronger effect on Y as body mass index (BMI) increases;
- X is only associated with Y among adults without a university degree;
- X is only associated with Y in older age groups;
- X increases risk in one group, but decreases risk in another group.

As an example, research has shown that personality traits such as neuroticism are associated with increased risk of psychiatric morbidity. For example, neuroticism is associated with increased risk of personality disorders, mood disorders, obsessive compulsive disorders and minor psychiatric morbidity. Other studies have suggested however, that socio-economic status (SES) may modify this risk. Put differently, the risk associated with personality traits might vary, depending on one's level of SES. Some traits might have stronger effects among low SES groups.

The data below are from the Health and Lifestyle Survey (1984), a representative sample of the UK population at the time. The analytic sample comprises 4570 participants with available data on personality traits, social class and psychiatric morbidity.

Neuroticism is considered the exposure of interest. High scores on neuroticism indicate a personality trait characterised by negative emotionality, anxiety, distress and worry. To obtain this score, participants completed the Eysenck Personality Inventory (EPI) which was used to create a neuroticism score. The scores were divided into tertiles (thirds) and the highest tertile are considered 'high neuroticism' in this exercise. The outcome of interest is being in the highest tertile of General Health Questionnaire-30 (GHQ-30) scores. The GHQ-30 measures minor psychiatric morbidity on a scale ranging from 30 to 120, derived from 30 questions (scored 0 to 3) which measure different aspects of this outcome. Participants were asked these question in relation to the past few weeks. Examples include: 'Have you recently … been able to concentrate on whatever you're doing?' and '… lost much sleep over worry?'

The effect modifier we want to evaluate is low SES, measured by having a manual occupational social class. Occupational social class was measured using the Registrar General system, which divided participants into six groups (I, II, III non-manual, III manual, IV, V). Manual social class (III manual, IV or V) is considered a potential effect modifier. It could also be considered an exposure, since we know that low SES is associated with psychiatric morbidity. For the purposes of this exercise however, we are interested in how it might change the relationship between neuroticism and GHQ-score. Chapters 13 and 14 will explain how to include two exposures and their interaction within the same statistical model. Here, we use a simplified approach which is to stratify groups according to the level of the effect modifier. That is, we will calculate the OR in non-manual and manual groups separately, determine if the OR is different in each group, and test whether any effect modification observed is significant. The process is similar to how we approached confounding. Essentially, we are breaking down the main 2 × 2 table into a set of smaller tables, one per group. The research question is, 'does low socio-economic status modify the association between neuroticism and minor psychiatric morbidity'? The data are shown in Table 6.2 for the whole analytic sample and for non-manual and manual groups separately.

First look at the crude OR for the combined group, the rightmost column at the bottom of the table. There is clearly a strong association between neuroticism and being in the worst GHQ tertile. Now look at the OR for manual social class groups and compare this to the OR for non-manual social class groups. The OR is stronger in manual groups. This could suggest that social class modifies the risk. The effect of neuroticism is stronger if you also have manual social class. Put differently, the combined effect of having manual social class and high neuroticism will increase your risk of minor psychiatric morbidity further. The OR is apparently different in each group, but are they significantly different?

We can test whether the ORs are significantly different using the chi-squared test for heterogeneity. If there was no effect modification, each of the stratum-specific ORs would be the same or nearly the same as the overall summary odds ratio. In the example above, the logic that follows is:

$$OR_{MH} = OR_{men} = OR_{women}$$

The chi-squared test is based on a weighted sum of squares of the differences between the odds ratios. By 'weighted' we mean that the test allows for the fact that the sample sizes are different in each stratum. The formula below uses V, which we encountered above when calculating the confidence intervals for the adjusted OR when looking at confounding.

$$\chi^2 = \sum \frac{(ad - OR_{MH} \times cb)^2}{OR_{MH} \times V \times n^2}, \quad d.f. = c - 1$$

In the equation, the calculations are performed on each stratum separately and then added together. This equation may look complex, but we can break it down into steps. Some of the steps will be familiar, because they are also used when we calculate confidence intervals for the adjusted OR (see above, steps 1, 2, 3 and 6 are also used below). Remember however that we are testing for significant effect modification, we are not adjusting for confounding. As discussed below, confounding and effect modification are quite different things.

Table 6.2 Data from the SES and psychiatric morbidity study

	Non-manual social class			Manual social class			Total		
	High GHQ	Low GHQ	Total	High GHQ	Low GHQ	Total	High GHQ	Low GHQ	Total
Highest tertile of neuroticism	397	317	714	535	330	865	932	647	1579
Lowest two tertiles of neuroticism	259	1174	1433	269	1289	1558	528	2463	2991
Total	656	1491	2147	804	1619	2423	1460	3110	4570
Stratum-specific ORs	$OR_{non-manual} = ad/bc$ $OR_{non-manual} = 5.68$			$OR_{manual} = ad/bc$ $OR_{manual} = 7.77$			$OR_{crude} = ad/bc$ $OR_{crude} = 6.72$		

Before starting, we need to calculate Q, R and V, because Q/R provides the adjusted OR and V provides the variance. These were steps 1, 2 and 3 above. Both are needed for chi-square test of heterogeneity.

$$Q = \sum \frac{ad}{n} = \frac{397 \times 1174}{2147} + \frac{535 + 1289}{2423} = 501.6954$$

$$R = \sum \frac{cb}{n} = \frac{259 \times 317}{2147} + \frac{269 \times 330}{2423} = 74.8772$$

$$V = \sum \frac{ghef}{n^2(n-1)} = \frac{656 \times 1491 \times 714 \times 1433}{2147^2(2147-1)} + \frac{804 \times 1619 \times 865 \times 1558}{2423^2(2423-1)} = 224.5343$$

$$\mathrm{OR}_{\mathrm{MH}} = \frac{Q}{R} = \frac{501.6954}{74.8772} = 6.7002$$

Having calculated Q, R and V, three additional steps are needed as shown in Table 6.3.

Since there are two groups, there is one degree of freedom (2–1=1). The chi-square statistic is 4.1132, which is significant at the $p < .05$ level with 1 degree of freedom. Therefore, we reject the null hypothesis that there is no heterogeneity in the odds ratios across the two strata (non-manual and manual social class). The association between neuroticism and minor psychiatric morbidity is different in the two strata (5.68 in the non-manual group, 7.77 in the manual group). The probability of attaining this result, if the null hypothesis was true, is very small.

The example shown above is intentionally a relatively simple one, in which we assumed there were no confounding factors, and there were only two strata. In reality, there may be one or more confounding factors and more than two strata. To take into account both confounding and effect modification, other statistical methods are usually deployed such as regression (Chapters 13 and 14).

Understanding the difference between confounding and effect modification

There is an important difference between stratification to control for confounding and stratification to evaluate effect modification. The modifier does not 'distort' the association between the exposure and the outcome, the modifier changes the association. The overall OR of 6.72 for both groups is broadly equivalent to the average effect for manual and non-manual groups. Confounding can produce distorted estimates which do not show the existence, correct size, or even correct direction of an effect. Researchers try to remove confounding as far as possible at the analysis stage. In contrast, effect modification can reveal estimates closer to the truth. Researchers try to identify effect modification and report this at the analysis stage. Confounding is a nuisance which we want to correct; effect modification is inherently interesting and we want to understand it.

Table 6.3 Chi-squared calculation

	Step 1	Step 2	Step 3
$OR_{MH} = 6.7002$ $V = 224.5343$	$(ad - OR_{MH} \times cb)^2$	$OR_{MH} \times V \times n^2$	$\chi^2 = \sum \dfrac{(ad - OR_{MH} \times cb)^2}{OR_{MH} \times V \times n^2}$
Non-manual social class	$= ((397 \times 1174) - 6.7002 \times (259 \times 317))^2$ $= ((466078) - 6.7002 \times (82103))^2$ $= 7061380612$	$= 6.7002 \times 101.1654176 \times 2147^2$ $= 3124544380$	$= \dfrac{(ad - OR_{MH} \times cb)^2}{OR_{MH} \times V \times n^2}$ $= \dfrac{7061380612}{3124544380}$ $= 2.2600$
Manual social class	$= ((535 \times 1289) - 6.7002 \times (269 \times 330))^2$ $= ((689615) - 6.7002 \times (88770))^2$ $= 8994292904$	$= 6.7002 \times 224.5343 \times 2147^2$ $= 4852916845$	$= \dfrac{(ad - OR_{MH} \times cb)^2}{OR_{MH} \times V \times n^2}$ $= \dfrac{8994292904}{4852916845}$ $= 1.8532$
Total			$= 2.2600 + 1.8532$ $= 4.1132$

The exercise below may help you understand the different between confounding and effect modification. It also illustrates an important point worth remembering – both confounding and effect modification can exist at the same time.

Box 6.1 Exercise: confounding and effect modification

The following hypothetical set of results (adapted from [40]) shows the relative risk (RR) of cigarette smoking and developing oral cancer, grouped by heavy alcohol drinking status. Use Table 6.4 to answer questions 1 to 4.

Table 6.4 Data for exercise on confounding and effect modification scenario

(A–D)	Heavy alcohol drinker (RR)	Non-heavy alcohol drinker (RR)	Combined alcohol drinking groups
(RR)			
A	4.0	1.0	2.0
B	4.0	4.0	1.0
C	4.0	2.0	1.0
D	4.0	4.0	4.0

1 Which scenario in Table 6.4 shows that heavy alcohol use is most likely to be a confounder but not an effect modifier?

2 Which scenario in the table shows that heavy alcohol use is most likely to be an effect modifier but not a confounder?

3 Which scenario in the table shows that heavy alcohol use is most likely to be neither a confounder nor an effect modifier?

4 Which scenario in the table shows that heavy alcohol use is most likely to be an effect modifier and a confounder?

Answers are given on the book website.

Mediating variables

Rarely does an exposure have a direct influence on a health outcome. In reality, exposures are connected to health outcomes through a series of different events. Exposures often influence physiological variables, and it is pathophysiological changes that actually cause disease, rather than the exposure itself. Nonetheless, we often simplify statistical models to consider only the exposure and the health outcome. Models should always be as simple as possible. In some situations however, it is necessary to illustrate which intermediate variable(s) connect an exposure with a health outcome.

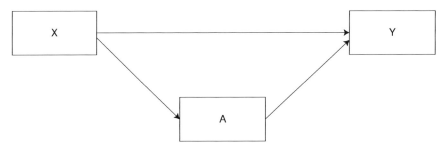

Figure 6.4 Mediating variables

Intermediate variables are called mediators, because they inter-mediate an association between an exposure (*X*) and an outcome (*Y*). Mediators can be physiological variables, but they could be health behaviours (e.g. smoking), psychosocial characteristics (e.g. mood, stress) among other things.

In the Figure 6.5 (adapted from [41], p.15), we can see that risk factors may exert their influence on health and disease through a complex chain of risks. There are several mediators, some of which are closer to the health outcome (more proximal) and some of which are further away (more distal). The risk factor could influence the outcome over many years, perhaps even decades. This kind of situation cannot be captured in a simple 2 × 2 table, where one exposure is associated with one outcome.

Consider a simple mediation model in which an exposure influences a health outcome, through a mediator. In Figure 6.5, childhood socio-economic status (SES; e.g. measured by the father's social class at birth) influences educational attainment, which influences self-rated health in adulthood in turn. The mediator (education) lies on the causal chain. People with higher childhood SES may be more likely to have better self-rated health in adulthood, *because* they obtain higher levels of education. This situation is entirely plausible, because we know that parental SES influences how long children stay in

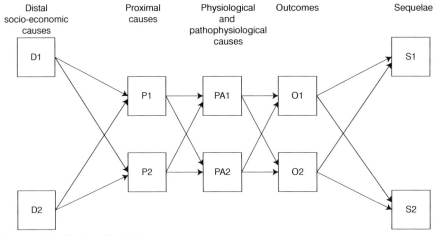

Figure 6.5 Chain of risk factors

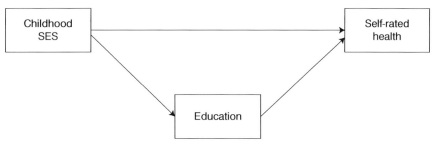

Figure 6.6 A simple mediation model

the education system for, and the qualifications they obtain. We also know that educational attainment is associated with better health outcomes. The arrows point from childhood SES to education, and from education to self-rated health, illustrating the proposed sequence of events. This situation is different from confounding. Confounding factors are illustrated with arrows that point to the exposure and to the outcome, implying that the confounder causes the exposure and the outcome (and hence the confounding or spurious association). In the mediation situation, the third variable is not a confounding factor. It is part of a real causal sequence.

Mediators are also known by other names, depending on the context. For example, they are often called mechanisms particularly when the meditator is a physiological/biological variable. Smoking is associated with lung cancer, but one of the key mechanisms is DNA damage in the lungs. Mediators are also called explanatory variables, because if they can be shown to mediate an association, they have explained the association. If we can show that X is associated with M (A in the Figure 6.6) and M with Y in turn, then we have explained why X is associated with Y (assuming that confounding is not present and the variables have been measured reliably and are valid). As we shall see below, traditional approaches to mediation analysis have focused on what happens to the X–Y association when the mediator is added to a statistical model. Finally, mediators are sometimes called 'causal confounders'. This is because mediators can produce an apparently confounded association between X and Y. Unlike confounding however, causal confounding occurs for a specific reason – the causal sequence.

The traditional approach to testing for mediation is called the Barron and Kenny [42] approach and involves linear regression, which is discussed in Chapter 13. We will consider the Barron and Kenny approach in that chapter. Briefly, researchers first establish that X and Y are associated. Then they establish that X and M are associated. Then they try to predict Y using both X and M. If X is no longer associated with Y when we use information about M to predict Y, then full mediation is said to have occurred. If X is still associated with Y even when M is considered, then partial mediation is said to have occurred. For now, it is worth thinking about why X and M might both be associated with Y. Sometimes however, X might have a direct association with Y which is not fully accounted for by the mediator. For example, childhood SES might influence health for reasons other than educational attainment. In this situation, we have partial mediation. To help clarify situations in which this happens, researchers distinguish between two types of effects: direct and indirect.

Direct effects are the association between X and Y that remains, after the mediator has been considered. As the name implies, we assume that X is partly causing Y, although some of the effect is transmitted by the mediator. The indirect effect is the pathway from X to M to Y. It is important to remember that direct and indirect pathways may exist, and often do exist. Statistical models to represent these kind of situations are beyond the scope of this book, but it is important to understand conceptually what full mediation (only an indirect effect exists) and partial mediation (direct and indirect effects exist) mean. It is also important to remember the distinction between confounding and mediation. It is the direction of the arrow between X and M that clarifies this distinction.

Antecedent variables

Antecedent variables (A in Figure 6.7) are variables that occur before the proposed exposure (X). A common situation in the health sciences is for researchers to claim to have found an association between X and Y, when in fact an unobserved antecedent variable is the 'true' exposure. In fact, we could re-label the antecedent as X, in which case the originally proposed exposure would then become a mediator.

Sometimes we cannot be sure which of the variables is the antecedent and which is the exposure. This is particularly problematic in cross-sectional studies or in prospective studies where both variables were measured at the same time. We might not know when each exposure actually occurred. For example, suppose that we measure educational attainment and a measure of 'confidence in academic ability' in a questionnaire, at the baseline of a prospective cohort study. We then follow participants to observe their subsequent health outcomes. Did the participant have stronger confidence in their ability because they had good educational attainment, or did prior confidence in academic ability influence their educational success?

Understanding antecedent variables depends on having information about them. This may not be available, which you should keep in mind when appraising the results of research studies. Without information about antecedent variables, we cannot rule out the possibility that earlier exposures

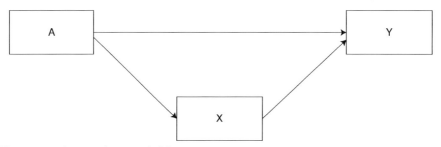

Figure 6.7 Antecedent variables

are the ones we should really be interested in. When critically appraising a paper, it is important to ask yourself if there might be antecedent variables which the authors have not considered. The importance of early life exposures is one of the reasons for the growth in popularity of life course approaches to health and disease, which consider sequences of events beginning in childhood, tracking participants through adolescence, adulthood and eventually old age. Such data are relatively rare, but quite a few studies have 'life course data' covering at least part of the life course. Examples of antecedent variables that you should keep in mind are:

- exposures earlier than birth, such as genetic factors;
- epigenetic effects (interactions between genes and environments, over several generations);
- prenatal exposures;
- early nutrition;
- parenting style;
- childhood SES;
- early educational exposures;
- occupational environments (e.g. asbestos);

Causal variables

If X is associated with Y, and this association is not confounded, modified or better explained by an antecedent variable, then it might be deemed a cause of Y. The temporal sequence must be clear, which is why prospective cohort studies provide better quality evidence about causality than cross-sectional observational studies. However, establishing the temporal sequence (X came before Y) is only one of several criteria which need to be met, before we can declare that X is a cause of Y. In this section we will consider how causality is evaluated.

The first step is to rule out alternative explanations for an association. Before determining if an association is causal, we have to rule out alternative possibilities:

1 the scenario has not been specified correctly; one or more third variables should be considered – are they confounders, mediators, effect modifiers or antecedents?

2 the association occurred by chance;

3 bias (see Appendix 8).

If these alternative explanations can be ruled out, the next step is to consider the nine Bradford Hill criteria for establishing causality. The Bradford Hill criteria comprise:

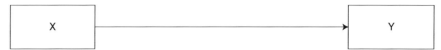

Figure 6.8 Causal variables

1 *Strength*: stronger associations between exposures and outcomes are more likely to be causal, assuming that they are not confounded.

2 *Consistency*: if an association is causal, then the exposure should be associated with the outcome consistently.

3 *Specificity*: if an association is causal, it should have mechanisms (mediators) that explain it. It follows that exposures should be associated with specific biological pathways and events, rather than general outcomes.

4 *Temporality*: the exposure should be known to occur before the outcome, as discussed above.

5 *Biological gradient*: sometimes called 'dose-response' association, a biological gradient implies that more exposure should lead to more harm. We should see that as exposure increases, so does the risk. We should not see the same risk, regardless of how much people were exposed.

6 *Biological plausibility*: the association should be plausible, usually meaning that there are biologically plausible mechanisms (mediators) to explain why the exposure and outcome are linked. These do not necessarily have to be shown in the same study, but a claim that an exposure causes a disease is more believable if plausible mechanisms exist. Having said that, we should not assume that just because mechanisms are (as yet) unknown, the association cannot be causal. It takes time to understand mechanisms fully, and there may be sufficiently strong evidence that an exposure is harmful, without knowing why it is harmful. Bradford Hill noted that what we think is biologically plausible 'depends upon the biological knowledge of the day' [43](p.10).

7 *Coherence*: the association should 'fit' with existing knowledge about a disease or a health problem. Coherence refers to conference with 'generally known facts of the natural history and biology of the disease' [43] (p.10).

8 *Experiment*: randomised controlled trials (Chapter 8) that assign one group an exposure/treatment are able to produce evidence that the exposure caused the outcome, because the randomisation process deals with known and unknown confounding factors. The two groups differ only in terms of the exposure. Observational studies (Chapter 9) however, cannot produce this kind of conclusion – there may be unknown confounding factors, even if the known confounding factors have been taken into consideration. It is often possible however, to supplement knowledge about an association discovered in a cohort study with evidence from experiments that show

how an exposure might cause the kinds of outcomes seen in observational data. Animal work for example, can be used to demonstrate 'proof of concept', or other lab-based experiments.

9 *Analogy*: analogy with similar exposures or similar diseases can help establish causality. For example, we would be more likely to expect drug X to cause Y if a similar drug also caused Y. Analogy involves finding something which is like the given thing in some way. For example, suppose that exposure A is like exposure B. Chemical M is in exposure A. Chemical N is in exposure B. So chemical M is like chemical N. This thought process is called analogical reasoning, and can be used to support causal inference.

It is not possible for any single study to satisfy all of these criteria. Consistency of an association, for example, can only be observed if we look at the results from several studies. We often have to appraise the totality of evidence from across the wider scientific literature. This is achieved through systematic reviews and meta-analysis, which are introduced in Chapter 7. As an example of an exposure that has been shown to be causal, consider cigarette smoking as a cause of lung cancer mortality. We can demonstrate that cigarette smoking meets all nine criteria:

1 *Strength*: Smoking is strongly associated with cancer. The risk of lung cancer mortality for smokers is around 15 times higher than for non-smokers [44], a large association.

2 *Consistency*: Smoking is consistently associated with lung cancer mortality. Smoking is associated with lung cancer mortality in different countries, in men and women, across different birth cohorts (generations), across the age range, and across all socio-economic groups [45]. This is clearly a highly consistent association. Bradford Hill was particularly keen on results that were similar but obtained in different ways (e.g. from different study designs), which is indeed seen in studies of smoking and cancer risk.

3 *Specificity*: Smoking is strongly associated with the different kinds of lung cancer [46], but less strongly associated with other kinds of cancer and with all-cause mortality risk. This is evidence that the association is more specific to biological pathways that are exposed to tobacco smoke. Specificity in the magnitude of the association points to a specific increase for lung cancer risk. When evaluating specificity of an association however, we have to keep in mind that diseases may have multiple causes (multi-causation, discussed below). This can make it difficult to draw strong conclusions about specificity, given that for example, lung cancer may occur for other reasons.

4 *Temporality*: In evaluating the association between smoking and subsequent lung cancer risk, smoking occurs earlier in time than the outcome (lung cancer).

5 *Biological gradient*: The relative risk of lung cancer increases with the number of cigarettes smoked [44]. Those exposed to more cigarettes have more risk. This is strong evidence for a 'dose-response' association.

6 *Biological plausibility*: It is biologically plausible that smoking increases lung cancer risk, because cigarettes contain more than 70 known carcinogens [45] that can cause DNA damage in the lung.

7 *Coherence*: Analysis of pathophysiological changes in lung tissue from smokers, and animal research showing how cigarette smoke affects skin tissue, are examples of evidence that is coherent with the smoking-lung cancer mortality association. So is the observation that lung cancer increased during the twentieth century as cigarette smoking increased.

8 *Experimental evidence*: Mice exposed to cigarette smoke have a higher risk of cancers compared to unexposed mice. Since only the exposure differed between these groups, this is good quality evidence that the cigarette smoke caused the cancers. We would not perform this kind of experiment with humans, but would expect the same results.

9 *Analogy*: Cigarette smoking is associated with lung cancer, and so are hand rolled cigarettes, pipes and cigars.

Bradford Hill concluded his article [43] by stressing that all research is incomplete. He said we should not ignore the data that we already do have, waiting until evidence is complete before taking action [43].

Necessary and sufficient causes

In Rothman's component causes model, [47, 48] a necessary cause is defined as a causal factor X which is necessary, but not sufficient, in order to produce an effect (e.g. exposure to the HIV virus is necessary but not sufficient for an individual to become HIV positive). A sufficient cause is a chain of events that will produce an effect (e.g. repeated exposure to an individual with HIV, repeated unprotected sexual intercourse, genetic susceptibility to HIV infection, absence of antiretroviral drugs). In this conceptual model, a cause is not a single entity but a set or chain of events (sufficient causes) that produce an effect. If one of the events is missing, the outcome will not happen.

Taking action before the cause is known and understood

Many people working in the applied health sciences, particularly public health, do not have the luxury of waiting even for good quality evidence – they have to act on the best quality evidence available, even if it lower down in the hierarchy of evidence than they would like. Arriving at the decision to interpret X as a cause always involves some subjectivity. If you decide that it is worth taking action based on the best available evidence to date, be sure that you are up to date with the evidence and be prepared to change your decision if required, as new data become available. Strategies for conducting reviews of the available literature are covered in Chapter 7.

Part III

Critical appraisal of existing research

7

Literature reviewing and database searching

Whether you work or intend to work in the health sciences, or become a health sciences researcher, regularly searching the existing published literature is essential. In this chapter, we will learn about major search tools used by health scientists, covering the two main databases which contain the majority of health sciences research (PubMed and PsycINFO). We will also look at methods for searching the literature systematically, and keeping good records of the searches you have made. Next, the chapter introduces social networking approaches to keeping on top of the literature and getting yourself organised, using CiteULike as an example. Finally, the chapter will show you how to import references into bibliographic software, using a popular program called EndNote.

Intended learning outcomes

By the end of this chapter you should be able to:

- understand the difference between narrative and systematic reviews;

- know what the stages of a systematic review are;

- design a systematic search strategy;

- find suitable medical subject headings (MeSH) for research articles;

- search PubMed and PsycINFO to identify published research papers on a topic;

- appreciate the need to search at least two databases;

- export references from your search into CiteULike;

- import references into bibliographic software (e.g. EndNote or Reference Manager).

Once you know how to search the literature to identify previous studies, you will be well-placed to start 'critically appraising' the literature, which is covered in the next three chapters. You will also be well-placed to design new research questions, which build on the work of others, adding new evidence for the scientific community to consider.

Narrative reviews of the literature

Narrative reviews of the literature are articles that describe several key studies in a particular field. These studies are selected by the author and are described in a 'narrative' without claiming to have searched the totality of articles available [2]. They may have been selected in 'pick and mix' fashion, because the author preferred these articles over others, or for various reasons. Narrative reviews can be very useful, particularly if you want a nice introduction to a topic. Textbooks can sometimes take the form of narrative reviews. Narrative reviews are subject to bias, however, because we usually do not know why the articles mentioned by the author were selected, in favour of other articles. What if one or more important articles were excluded from the review, for reasons unknown? Systematic reviews address this problem.

Systematic reviews of the literature

Conducting a systematic review of the literature will help you identify:

- the relevant studies on a topic;
- the best quality studies;
- a set of studies selected without bias, where possible;
- a set of studies that another researcher could reproduce, if they used the same methods as you.

The stages of a systematic review are:

- clarify the research question;
- conduct a scoping search;
- create and refine a set of search terms;
- choose which databases you should search;
- search the databases;
- export references into bibliographic software;
- identify and remove duplicates;
- remove references which are clearly unsuitable or 'off topic';
- save the 'high quality' list of references in another file;
- retrieve the references;
- read the articles;
- search the reference lists of the articles you retrieved;
- search for other articles which have cited the articles in your list;

- report your search, when it was conducted, what you found;
- optionally, conduct a meta-analysis of existing findings
  - meta-analysis does not necessarily follow a systematic review, but often does. Meta-analysis is discussed in the chapter on other research designs.

The Cochrane Collaboration have produced a manual (*The Cochrane Handbook for Systematic Reviews of Interventions* http://www.cochrane.org/training/cochrane-handbook) which instructs researchers how to conduct a full-scale and high-systematic review (see Chapter 6 of the *Cochrane Handbook*), often considered the 'gold standard' (best quality) for a systematic review. For most student projects, a systematic review of this standard is rarely required. It is important however, to decide how systematic you want your review to be. Be guided by your course requirements and your supervisors – and how much time you have. If you are searching a topic that is relatively novel or under-researched, searching the literature systematically might only take a few weeks or months. If you struggle to find many articles at all on your topic, you may even have to expand your search to make it less specific. If you are searching a topic that is very broad and is well-researched, with a large literature, a systematic review could take months or even years. In this situation, you may want to refine your search to make it more specific.

Even if your review is purely for a student project, and you have no intention of publishing your review, it is important to keep good records throughout the entire process, so make sure that you keep notes along the way. Ideally, you should be able to present your review as a study flow diagram. Figure 7.1 is an example, reproduced from the *Cochrane Handbook*.

If you decide to publish your literature review, which is something you may want to consider at a later date, do consult the Preferred Reporting Items for Systematic Reviews and Meta-Analyses (PRISMA) guidelines first (see www.prisma-statement.org). This is a minimum set of guidelines that people will expect you to have followed, in conducting your review.

- Researchers frequently rely on less formalised methods of reviewing the literature. Examples of strategies often used are:
- *Narrative reviews*: these have been described ealier.
- *Searching Google and Google Scholar*. This is particularly useful at the 'scoping' stage of a review before you decide to approach the literature systematically.
- *Grey literature*. Research which is not peer-reviewed and published in traditional academic outlets; examples include research conducted by charities or voluntary/community sector organisations. Grey literature databases are available (e.g. www.opengrey.eu, www.ntis.gov, www.greynet.org).

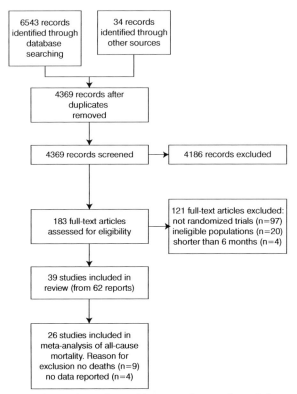

Figure 7.1 Systematic review flow diagram (reproduced from the *Cochrane Handbook,* Figure 11.2.a)

- *Journals.* Reading journals of particular interest to the researcher; for example, if you work in nursing you may regularly read nursing journals, where research in nursing will be published. As you become familiar with a topic, you will start to learn which journals tend to publish research on that topic. Avoid relying on this approach however, because restricting your reading to a narrow set of journals can mean that you miss other useful publication outlets.

- *Attending academic conferences.* This is an excellent way to keep up to date with the newest research in your area, but be careful – the findings should always be interpreted as provisional and have usually not undergone peer review at this stage.

- *Word of mouth.* This is obviously not a reliable or systematic way to identify existing research, but occasionally our peers can be a useful source of information. Talking to people who work in your area, particularly if they have expertise on the same topic, can help you retrieve sources that might otherwise have been missed.

- *Edited books.* Some researchers publish excellent work in book chapters, providing overviews and narrative reviews of an area.

- *Textbooks*. Textbooks can be nice comprehensive introductions to a field, providing a good range of references to existing research. They date quickly however, and many are not updated regularly. Consider using text books as a starting point, to familiarise yourself with a new field or area of study. You must however, read more recent papers on a topic, particularly if you plan to conduct your own research in order to add something new to the evidence base.

- *Social networking websites*. such as CiteULike or Academia.edu (see below).

The methods above all have their uses, but none of them should be relied upon if you want to conduct a thorough review of the literature. Think of these methods as ways to complement a literature review, or ways in which to extend your knowledge even further. All literature searching should involve at least some systematic elements.

Before you start

Before searching the literature, have a clear research question in mind. For example, use the PICO acronym in order to clarify your research question (see Table 7.1):

- *Patient/population*. What is the population you are interested in?

- *Intervention (or exposure)*. What is the intervention (for trials and other intervention studies) or the exposure (in epidemiological studies such as cohort designs)?

- *Control group*. What is the control group or reference group?

- *Outcome*. What is the outcome variable?

Your research question needs to be specific enough to identify a manageable set of articles to read, but sensitive enough to ensure that you do not exclude too many articles from your search.

Next, make some tables that will help you keep good records throughout your literature review. You may want to update your search in the future, or be asked to show how you obtained your search results. For these reasons, detailed tables of what you did, and when you did it, are useful; Table 7.2 shows an example.

Searching the literature with PubMed

PubMed is a popular web-based search tool for searching the medical literature (published papers or manuscripts 'in press' which are nearly published). From 1996, access to MEDLINE was made public through a search tool known as PubMed. PubMed is a web-based retrieval system. Its key features are:

Table 7.1 Using PICO to clarify research questions

Example research questions	P Patient/ population	I Intervention	C Control group	O Outcome	Comments
Do adult patients with diabetes have better glycaemic control if they receive text message reminders about monitoring blood sugar?	Adult diabetes patients	Text messages	Treatment as usual	Glycaemic control	This is a clear research question
Is diet linked to health?	Not clear	Diet. Not clear which aspect of diet.	Not clear	Not clear – what aspect of health (physical/mental)?	This research question is far too broad
Do children with both Munchausen and Prader-Willi syndrome experience less weight gain if they are refused food when presenting at hospitals in Yorkshire?	Children with both Munchausen and Prader-Willi syndrome (both are rare disorders) in Yorkshire	Refusal of food at hospitals?	Children not refused food at hospitals in Yorkshire	Weight	This research question is too specific. Both diseases are rare. It is even rarer to have both diseases.

Table 7.2 Records of searches in a literature review

Database	Dates covered	Date searched	Search terms	Detail	Results	My notes
PubMed	01/01/1952+	19/06/13	"narcissistic personality disorder"	"narcissistic personality disorder "[All Fields] AND (Review[ptyp] AND ("1952/01/01" [PDAT] : "3000/12/31" [PDAT]))	29	DSM-I published 1952
PsycINFO	1987 to June Week 2 2013	19/06/13	"narcissistic personality disorder"	exp Narcissistic Personality Disorder/	1111	Used the OVID search interface.

- more than 22 million articles are indexed;

- some books are indexed;

- new articles 'in press' or still in production are included;

- worldwide coverage (although more than 80 per cent of articles are in English or have an English abstract)

Using medical subject headings (MeSH)

Medical subject headings (MeSH) are used to help organise PubMed articles. They are very similar to 'keywords' that you might use when searching the web, but are more formally organised. MeSH are described as controlled vocabulary, controlled in the sense that these words are used consistently throughout the database, to help avoid confusion. For example, if you wanted to search for articles about the term 'hospital addiction', the appropriate MeSH term is 'Munchausen syndrome', a disorder characterised by fabrication of symptoms in order to receive repeated hospital care unnecessarily.

This returns the following MeSH headings, which are the standardised search terms (controlled vocabulary) you should use in PubMed:

- Munchausen Syndrome

- Hospital-Addiction Syndrome

- Syndrome, Hospital-Addiction

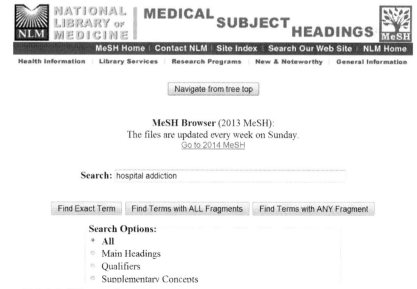

Figure 7.2 MeSH search page

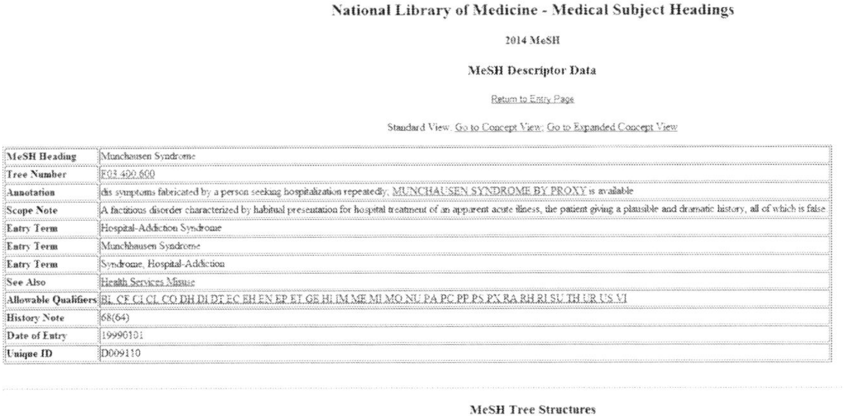

National Library of Medicine - Medical Subject Headings

2014 MeSH

MeSH Descriptor Data

Return to Entry Page

Standard View; Go to Concept View; Go to Expanded Concept View

MeSH Heading	Munchausen Syndrome
Tree Number	F03.420.600
Annotation	dis symptoms fabricated by a person seeking hospitalization repeatedly; MUNCHAUSEN SYNDROME BY PROXY is available
Scope Note	A factitious disorder characterized by habitual presentation for hospital treatment of an apparent acute illness, the patient giving a plausible and dramatic history, all of which is false
Entry Term	Hospital-Addiction Syndrome
Entry Term	Munchausen Syndrome
Entry Term	Syndrome, Hospital-Addiction
See Also	Health Services Misuse
Allowable Qualifiers	BL CF CI CL CO DH DI DT EC EH EN EP ET GE HI IM ME MI MO NU PA PC PP PS PX RA RH RI SU TH UR US VI
History Note	68(64)
Date of Entry	19990101
Unique ID	D009110

MeSH Tree Structures

Figure 7.3 Searching MeSH

A row will appear called 'Annotation' which provides a definition and also suggests the related term 'Munchausen syndrome by proxy'. Clicking on this link explains that symptoms can be fabricated by parents for their children.

The row 'See also' can also be quite useful, because it suggests other related terms that might interest you. Here, the term 'Health Services Misuse' is provided.

MeSH has a hierarchical structure, which you can learn more about from the MeSH website (www.nlm.nih.gov/mesh).

Some key points about how PubMed uses MeSH terms:

- If you search a MeSH term, all narrower terms are automatically included (called 'explosion').

- If you search a MeSH term that appears elsewhere in the hierarchy, all narrower terms from each instance will be included.

There are many other useful features of PubMed, and it is worth investing some time in learning how to use them. There are tutorials available on the PubMed website or on YouTube.

Designing a systematic search strategy

It is helpful to search databases systematically, rather than chopping and changing various keywords you happen to think might capture the literature you are interested in. Articles are often, but not always, indexed using key words and in the case of PubMed, MeSH headings. It is useful to spend some time thinking about which key words you should search with.

If you enter a set of terms into the search field on PubMed, it will try to match what you enter into the search field to its own lists. PubMed will attempt to match what you have entered sequentially:

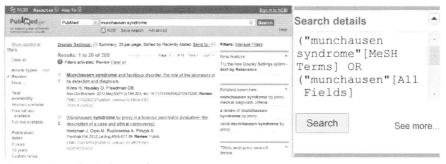

Figure 7.4 PubMed search

- MeSH headings
- journal
- author names

For example, if you enter 'Munchausen syndrome', a match will be found to the MeSH term for this disorder. It will also look for combinations of 'Munchausen' and 'syndrome' in any field, and the phrase 'Munchausen syndrome' in any field. In this example, a match is made to a MeSH heading and so PubMed stops there – it will not continue looking at journal or author names. If it cannot find a MeSH heading match or find the term in other fields, it will try looking for journals then authors.

The search results are displayed in the main PubMed window, and the search details box provides the exact syntax used to retrieve this list of articles:
"munchausen syndrome" [MeSH Terms] OR ("munchausen" [All Fields] AND "syndrome" [All Fields]) OR "munchausen syndrome" [All Fields]

To the left, you can filter the results according to the type of article (e.g. review articles only, recent articles only).

This can be a useful starting point, particularly at the scoping stage of a review, but ideally you should design a systematic search string. This involves selecting relevant search terms and combining them with Boolean operators.

Boolean operators

Databases including PubMed use Boolean operators in order to specify the relationship between search terms.

- AND specifies that both terms must be present
- OR specifies that either term must be present
- NOT specifies that the second term is not present (but the first term is present)

Table 7.3 Using Boolean operators in search strings

Search string	Results
Stroke	~26,000
Ischemic Attack, Transient	~1600
stroke OR Ischemic Attack, Transient	~27,000
stroke AND Ischemic Attack, Transient	~900
stroke NOT Ischemic Attack, Transient	~25,000

~=around this figure, which is likely to have increased since time of writing.

You should become familiar with these Boolean operators, because they help you to create systematic search strings. Your searches will be more specific, more relevant and more manageable if you use clearly thought-out operators to connect your search strings. Consider this example, using Boolean operators to combine 'stroke' with 'Ischemic Attack, Transient' (the MeSH term for transient ischemic attack) in different ways:

In general, the operator OR will result in a larger number of results. For this reason, AND and NOT are useful if you want a more specific search. The OR operator results in a more sensitive, but less specific search. Depending on the topic you are searching for, you will have to think carefully about how to combine search terms in order to balance sensitivity with specificity in your search.

An alternative to using AND to specify that two terms should appear together, is to force them together using quotation marks. Quotation marks tell PubMed to treat the terms as a phrase. For example 'intermittent explosive disorder' might return around 20 results, whereas treating these terms separately might return more than 800. You might want to try using terms without quotation marks first, before restricting the results to include your phrase.

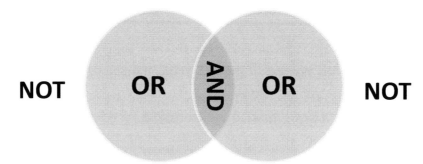

Figure 7.5 Boolean operator results

Searching the literature with PsycINFO

Although PsycINFO is a database of psychology research, a large amount of research relevant to the health sciences can be found here. For example, you will find research about cognitive function, health behaviours, theories of behaviour change, community psychology, sexual behaviour and social marketing approaches to behaviour change. Some of the papers in PsycINFO are also indexed by PubMed, but by no means all of them. The journal *Intelligence*, for example, does not currently appear on PubMed, but does contain research about epidemiology, cognitive function and dementia. It is important however, not to rely on a single database when searching the literature. The study described below illustrates why.

PsycINFO has several attractive features for health scientists:

- coverage begins in 1887
- it uses controlled vocabulary for easier matching between search terms and key words
- books, book chapters and dissertations are included, not only journal articles
- covers behavioural, social and psychological aspects of health
- has over 1.5 million entries (although compared to PubMed, this is relatively few!)

PsycINFO is often, but not always, accessed through the OVID interface. Check with your librarian or information services support team to find out how you can access PsycINFO.

Searching PsycINFO

In this example, we will learn how to use PsycINFO to identify articles and book chapters for a research question 'Are sedentary behaviours in adolescence associated with common mental disorders?' Using the PICO acronym, we can separate this into three sets of key words that might be worth searching.

- *Population* adolescents.
- *Intervention/exposure*: sedentary behaviours (this is an epidemiological or observational research question, not an intervention study.
- *Control*: this is not applicable; sedentary behaviours are the exposure, so the unexposed group (equivalent to control group) are simply those with lower levels of sedentary behaviour.
- *Outcome*: common mental disorders, sometimes called minor psychiatric morbidity; this refers to symptoms of anxiety, depression, obsessive compulsive disorder and panic disorder.

Table 7.4 Using PsycINFO search terms

Sedentary behaviours (exposure)	AND	Adolescents (population)	AND	Common mental disorder (outcome)
sedentary behavio*		adolescen*		depress*
television viewing		boys		anxi*
screen-based media		child*		psychological distress
inactivity		girls		mood
computer		schoolage		affective
video		teenage		phobia
screen time		youth		ocd
				obsessive compulsive disorder
				panic
				dysthymia
				mental disorder
				psychiatric morbidity

Before we begin our search, it can be helpful to make a list of all the synonyms for each set. Use an asterisk to indicate that all terms starting with the letters in the word should be included. For example, depress* would include depression, depressive and depressed.

To get started, find the link to PsycINFO on your library's website. Often, it can be found in an alphabetical list. Click on the link to open the search interface.

PsycINFO is often provided by the OVID interface, but not always, so please check with your institution if the examples shown here differ substantially from what you see.

In OVID, PsycINFO, it is best to search for each set separately and then combine the results using AND to reduce the number of results. Because the term 'computer' might include computer-assisted interviews, a method used in a study rather than the topic of investigation, the keyword NOT is used to exclude interview from the results.

We will limit the search to results that have an abstract of the research available, human rather than animal studies and English language studies.

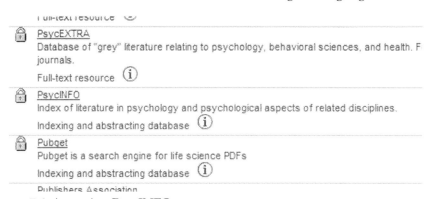

Figure 7.6 Accessing PsycINFO

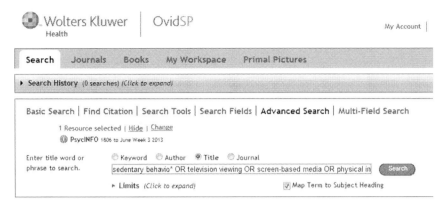

Figure 7.7 PsycINFO search page

These three sets of words can be combined as follows. Select the 'Title' radio button and tick the box 'Map Term to Subject Heading'. This will focus the search to ensure that sedentary behaviours, adolescence and common mental disorder all appear in the title. Mapping the term to subject headings will ask OVID to match our keywords to other subject headings we might have missed.

Search 1. sedentary behavio* OR television viewing OR screen-based media OR physical inactivity OR computer OR video OR screen time OR sitting time (Figure 7.7)

Enter the search terms, then click on 'Search' to run the search (Figure 7.8).

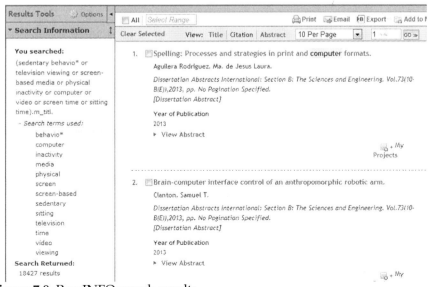

Figure 7.8 PyscINFO search results

The search returned 18,427 results, shown on the left hand side under 'Search Information'. The results themselves are shown in the main area of the screen. Obviously this is too many articles to read as part of a literature review, but remember that we have only searched for one of three parts of our search terms. The next step is to search for the second set of terms. OVID will automatically save the first search, so you can go ahead and enter the second set straight away, then click 'Search' again.

Search 2. adolescen* OR boys OR child* OR girls OR schoolage OR teenage OR youth

This produced 341,873 results. Obviously, these populations are commonly studied by psychologists and this has resulted in a large number of entries in the database. Continue with the third set of terms.

Search 3. depress* OR anxi* OR psychological distress OR mood OR affective OR phobia OR ocd OR obsessive compulsive disorder OR panic OR dysthymia OR mental disorder OR psychiatric morbidity

This produced 147,516 results.

The actual searches conducted by OVID PsycINFO are shown in the Search History. Scroll to the top of the screen to 'Search History', and click on the blue area to see them (Figure 7.9).

The term m_titl means that the search is restricted to titles and that terms are mapped to subject headings (Figure 7.10).

Having conducted three separate searches, we can now combine them with Boolean logic, to make the search more focused. This will reduce the number of results, because we are asking PsycINFO to return results containing all three of our searches. Tick the three boxes next to searches 1, 2 and 3. Then click 'And' to the right of 'Combine selections with' (Figure 7.11).

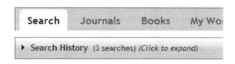

Figure 7.9 PyscINFO search history tab

	# ▲	Searches	Results	Search Type	Actions
☑	1	(sedentary behavio* or television viewing or screen-based media or physical inactivity or computer or video or screen time or sitting time).m_titl.	18427	Advanced	Display More ≫
☑	2	(adolescen* or boys or child* or girls or schoolage or teenage or youth).m_titl.	341873	Advanced	Display More ≫
☑	3	(depress* or anxi* or psychological distress or mood or affective or phobia or ocd or obsessive compulsive disorder or panic or dysthymia or mental disorder or psychiatric morbidity).m_titl.	147516	Advanced	Display More ≫

Figure 7.10 PsycINFO search history page

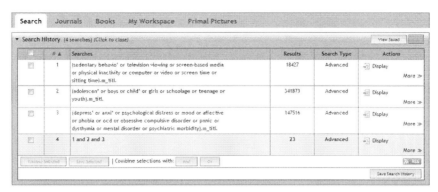

Figure 7.11 Combining PsycINFO search results

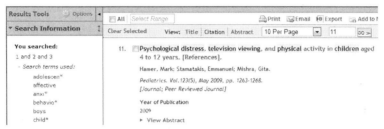

Figure 7.12 PsycINFO search: result 11

19. ☐ Effects of violent versus nonviolent **video** games on **children's** arousal, aggressive **mood**, and positive **mood**. [References].

Fleming, Michele J; Rickwood, Debra J.

Journal of Applied Social Psychology. Vol.31(10), Oct 2001, pp. 2047-2071.
[Journal; Peer Reviewed Journal]

Year of Publication
2001
▸ View Abstract

Figure 7.13 PsycINFO search: result 19

This search combined searches 1 to 3 in a new search, resulting in 23 articles. Many however, are obviously not relevant to our research question. This is clear when looking at the articles which are retrieved. The search has picked up several studies looking at 'computer anxiety' in children, which is not what we are interested in. Result number 11 does look relevant (Figure 7.12)

Result number 19 could also be relevant (Figure 7.13).

Given that our search of PsycINFO produced only two articles, we might want to consider searching other databases, particularly PubMed. Although the research literature on sedentary behaviours in adolescence and common mental disorders is quite small, we should not conclude that there are only two studies based on this single search.

Search tips for PsycINFO

- Use wildcards to replace one letter. For example, able# would find abler and ables but not ablest.

- If you select the title button, you can search for a title of a paper, book, book chapter or dissertation.

- If you select the author button, you can search for all entries by author last name.

- If you search for a journal, it helps to know the full journal name, because if you enter one word, only the journals beginning with that word will be retrieved. For example, Health Psychology would retrieve *Health Psychology* but not the *British Journal of Health Psychology*.

- You can limit your search according to the following: age, date, methodology, population, publication type.

- You can export your results to bibliographic software such as EndNote or Reference Manager.

- Remember that you should always search at least two databases.

- If you have too few results, your search may be too specific.

- Additional to a search, look at the references cited in the articles that you read. Did your search miss any of these references?

- Look at any articles citing articles you retrieve. These are displayed by many search interfaces, including Web of Knowledge and Google Scholar. This can be a useful way to identify relevant articles you might have missed, particularly those which are relatively new.

Other databases to consider searching

Although PubMed and PsycINFO are a good place to start, take a look at some of the many other databases of health research available.

- *Cochrane Library*: this is an excellent resource for research on efficacy and effectiveness of interventions or treatments. Systematic reviews are included in the Cochrane Library, as are 'Cochrane Reviews' which are considered the best quality quantitative research in the hierarchy of evidence.

- *Current Index to Nursing & Allied Health Literature (CINAHL)*: this database includes primarily nursing research, but also disciplines allied to medicine, complementary medicine, consumer health.

- *EMBASE*: this covers biomedical and pharmacological research, with a slightly more European emphasis than PubMed.

- *Google Scholar*: Google Scholar can be very useful because it can find articles, book chapters and books on a topic. The search results look very similar to an academic database search, rather than a traditional Google search. It claims to cover all scholarly literature. You can also look at citations to publications and create your own author profile.

- *Grey Literature Network Service (GreyNet):* this is a collection of 'grey literature' which includes research not published in traditional academic outputs. Grey literature can sometimes be a useful supplement to peer-reviewed academic articles, although you should appraise its quality carefully. The voluntary and community sector often produce good-quality research which they do not submit for publication in academic journals [49]. This does not mean that you should ignore the research, but it does mean that it has not undergone the formal peer review process.

- *Science Direct*: this is not a database as such, but an 'interface' which allows you to search for articles and access .pdf versions of documents where available. Some researchers find it quite useful.

- *Web of Science*: this is a popular database which includes science, social science and arts/humanities research. There is considerable overlap with PsycINFO but Web of Science does not include book chapters.

Many of these databases require a licence or subscription, so you should check with your institution to see if you are able to access them.

The need to search more than one database

A team of researchers who were planning to conduct systematic reviews for the Cochrane Collaboration decided to do a study in order to find out which psychiatry journals were indexed by which databases
Initially, they checked a resource called the Ulrich's Periodicals Directory for any journals relating to psychiatry or neurology. Although 122 journals were found to be captured by four popular databases, several journals were only found in one database (7 in MEDLINE, 25 in BIOSIS, 50 in EMBASE, 94 in PsycLIT – now PsycINFO). The degree of overlap between four databases is shown in Figure 7.14. The conclusion from this study was that relying on one database would exclude many psychiatry journals. In general, you should search at least two databases and ideally more than two, if you have time. This is particularly important in the health sciences, which often involves several disciplines, with research published in many different outlets. The example above involved just one discipline (psychiatry) – and yet journals publishing psychiatry research were spread across four different databases. Higher-impact and more well-known journals are more likely to be captured in several databases. The authors of this study, for example, found that the *American Journal of Psychiatry* was indexed in over 40 abstracting or indexing services.

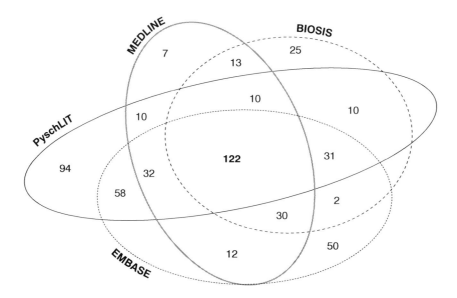

Figure 7.14 Overlap of BIOSIS, EMBASE, MEDLINE and PsychLIT for psychiatry journals (adapted from [50])

Social networking approaches to searching the literature

This section introduces a popular social networking tool which you may find useful when searching the literature, called CiteULike.

CiteULike

Increasingly, students and researchers work in multiple locations using different PCs, laptops and other devices. Storing all your references in one place can become difficult. To help you stay organised, one option is to store them on the web or the cloud, so that your databases are available from any location. CiteULike is one example of a web-based library that you can personalise and share with others (see www.citeulike.org).

CiteULike allows you to install browser buttons, so that a paper you find can be quickly added to your library, stored online. The service is compatible with many journals, and with Amazon, allowing you to quickly store articles and books in your own online library. If you look carefully, you can sometimes see a CiteULike button on a journal website itself. The example below is from the *British Journal of Health Psychology*, where you can quickly add a paper to your CiteULike library by clicking on the blue CiteULike button (to the right of 'Share').

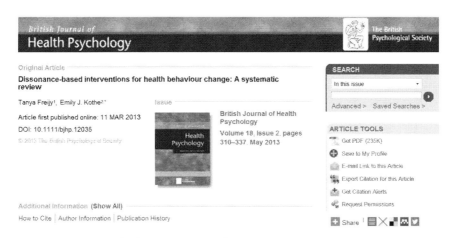

British Journal of
Health Psychology

Original Article

Dissonance-based interventions for health behaviour change: A systematic review

Tanya Freijy[1], Emily J. Kothe[2*]

Issue

Article first published online: 11 MAR 2013

DOI: 10.1111/bjhp.12035

© 2013 The British Psychological Society

British Journal of Health
Psychology
Volume 18, Issue 2, pages
310–337, May 2013

Figure 7.15 CiteULike button on a web page

You can organise your library according to keywords called tags. The tags are displayed in a tag cloud, with larger words for the tags you use more frequently. This provides you and others with a visual representation of your research interests. The tag cloud is useful because when you click on a tag, you will see all of your papers on this topic as a list. Similarly, you get a tag cloud for the authors you read most frequently. The tag cloud in Figure 7.16 is from the author's library (www.citeulike.org/user/gareth/tags). CiteULike tag clouds are public. By tagging articles with key words, you are helping other people find articles that might interest them. They have lots of articles tagged with cardiovascular, change, correlates, depression, health, immunity, longitudinal and measurement, for example. This tells you that this CiteULike user probably has research interests on psychobiology and cardiovascular health. If you go to their library online, you can click on these key words to see what articles have been tagged and stored. Similarly, other people can view your library, so by tagging articles you are helping others to find articles that might interest them.

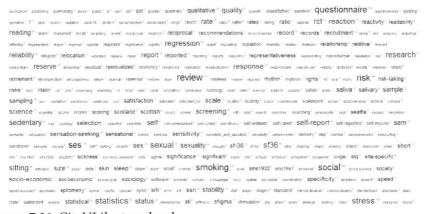

Figure 7.16 CiteULike tag cloud

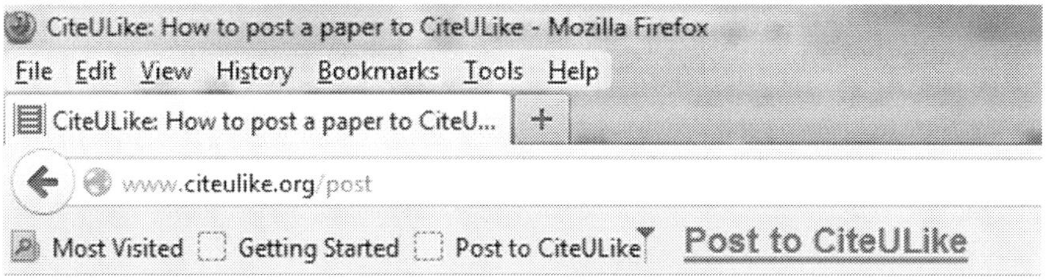

Figure 7.17 CiteULike bookmark link in Firefox

Getting started with CiteULike

To get started, sign up at www.citeulike.org and choose a username. Then install a CiteULike browser button on your browser, following the instructions on the CiteULike website (www.citeulike.org/post). If using the Firefox browser, for example, find the link 'Post to CiteULike', click and drag this to the bookmarks toolbar (below the address bar, as shown Figure 7.17) and then let go. A button labelled 'Post to CiteULike' should now be installed.

You may want to install browser buttons on more than one of your devices, but your account will be the same on every device. All your references will be stored in one place.

How to upload a paper to CiteULike

If the journal website has a CiteULike button, click the button. If not, click the button you have installed on your browser ('Post to CiteULike'). You will be taken to a page with the heading 'New Article: where would you like to file it?' (see Figure 7.18). If not, the journal may not be compatible with CiteULike. Check the CiteULike website and blog for information about which journals are currently compatible.

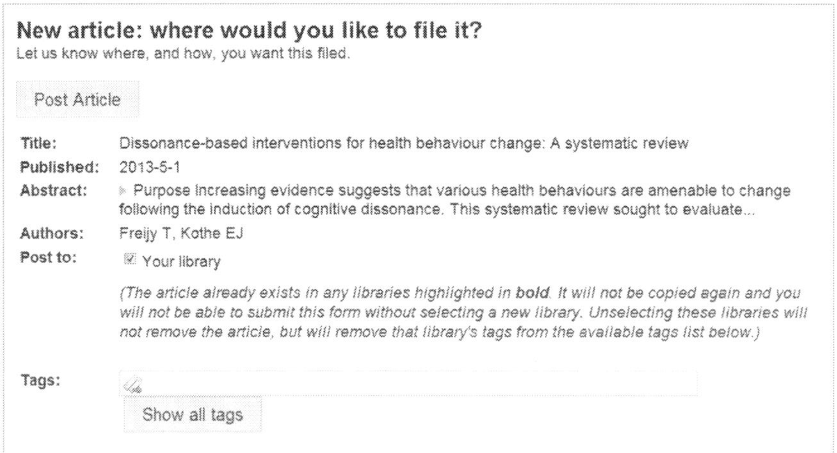

Figure 7.18 CiteULike new article page

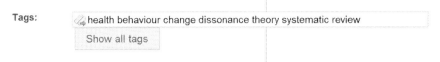

Figure 7.19 Tagging a CiteULike entry

In most cases, the article title, date, abstract and authors will have been automatically extracted for you. You may have to fill some of these fields in manually. In all cases, you should choose tags to help you find this article in your CiteULike library in future. Enter each tag, separated by commas (Figure 7.19).

The tags chosen for this article are: health, behaviour, change, dissonance, theory, systematic, review. Obviously, you need to choose tags that describe the article you want to store in your own library.

A really nice feature of CiteULike is the ability to upload and store .pdf versions of articles, and access these from anywhere. This avoids the need to keep paper or electronic copies of articles in several locations, because you always know that your CiteULike library has everything. There is an option to share .pdfs of your articles with other CiteULike users, but do check for any copyright or other restrictions before doing this. Often, publishers request that you do not circulate .pdfs of journal articles. They are usually restricted to your own use. You can upload a .pdf of the article by clicking on 'Choose File' under 'Attachment'. Finally, when you are ready to add the article to your library, click on 'Post Article'.

You may be wondering why CiteULike is considered a social network. This is because other people can see your tag cloud, and you can identify research interests shared by other people. People who read the same papers as you are likely to have similar research interests. In time, they may become colleagues, friends or competitors (or all three)! It can sometimes be handy to see what other people are reading, to keep up to date with the literature.

How to export an item from your CiteULike library

You may want to export articles or books from your CiteULike library to bibliographic software, such as EndNote (introduced later in the chapter). To do this, find the article you want to export from your library, then click on the 'Export' button.

You will then be shown a series of options for exporting the article details (Figure 7.21). If you are using Endnote or Reference Manager, you should click on 'RIS'. This will download the details. Click on the file that is downloaded to automatically store the reference in your bibliographic software.

To summarise, CiteULike allows you to store articles that you have found, tag them, store details of the articles in your own online library, store .pdfs of the articles themselves, and export them to bibliographic software. Your library, but not the .pdfs, are automatically shared with other users.

| Delete | Edit | Copy | Duplicate | Posts | Blog | Share | Export | Citation | Find Similar |

Figure 7.20 CiteULike toolbar

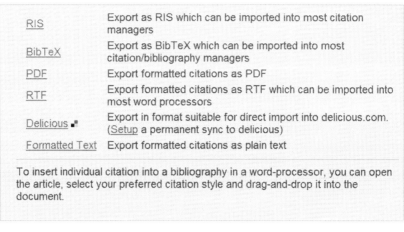

RIS	Export as RIS which can be imported into most citation managers
BibTeX	Export as BibTeX which can be imported into most citation/bibliography managers
PDF	Export formatted citations as PDF
RTF	Export formatted citations as RTF which can be imported into most word processors
Delicious	Export in format suitable for direct import into delicious.com. (Setup a permanent sync to delicious)
Formatted Text	Export formatted citations as plain text

To insert individual citation into a bibliography in a word-processor, you can open the article, select your preferred citation style and drag-and-drop it into the document.

✔ **Dissonance-based interventions for health behaviour change: A systematic review**
Br J Health Psychol, Vol. 18, No. 2. (1 May 2013), pp. 310-337, doi:10.1111/bjhp.12035
by Tanya Freijy, Emily J. Kothe
posted to behaviour change dissonance health review systematic theory by JamesWatson keyed Freijy2013Dissonancebased on 2013-11-07 13:30:04
★★/ along with 1 person
▓ Abstract ▓ Copy

Figure 7.21 CiteULike export options

Bibliographic software

EndNote

EndNote and Reference Manager are two popular bibliographic software packages (others are available) which will help you organise your literature review, keep a record of your references, and when you get to the writing stage, create a reference list for your thesis or manuscript. Check with your information support specialist, librarian or IT support team, to find out what software is available at your institution. Reference Manager is very similar to EndNote, but EndNote is generally more widely available at universities. For this reason, the examples shown below refer to EndNote.

References can be exported from PubMed, Web of Knowledge and many online journals, into EndNote. From EndNote, you can identify and remove duplicates. You can also type in your own references (e.g. books, book chapters, reports). Usefully, EndNote integrates with MS Word, so that reference lists can be generated automatically.

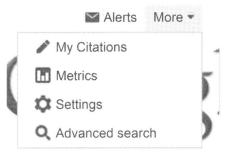

Figure 7.22 Google Scholar menu

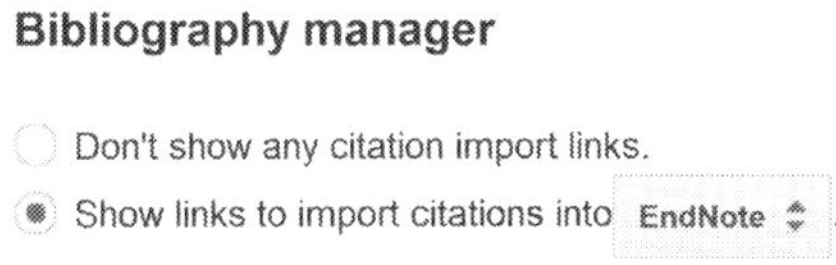

Bibliography manager

○ Don't show any citation import links.

◉ Show links to import citations into EndNote ⇕ .

Figure 7.23 Google Scholar Bibliography Manager

Exporting from Google Scholar to EndNote

Click on the settings symbol which can be found on the top right of Google Scholar (Figure 7.22).

Under Scholar Settings > Bibliography Manager, select the 'Show links to import citation into' button, then choose 'EndNote' (Figure 7.23).

Next time you conduct a search on Google Scholar, you will now see the option to export to EndNote ('Import into EndNote') for each reference retrieved (Figure 7.24).

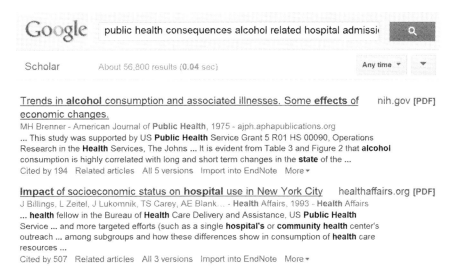

Figure 7.24 Google Scholar search results

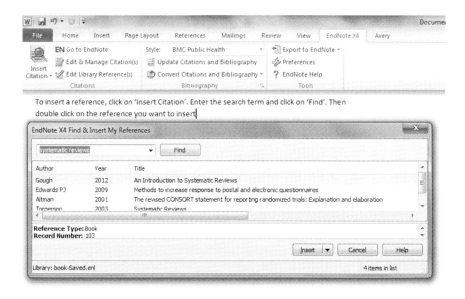

Figure 7.25 Inserting a citation using EndNote

Cite while you write

As mentioned above, when you get to the stage of writing your literature review, thesis, or manuscript, EndNote can help. You can insert references automatically and it will generate the reference list for you. Open MS Word and the EndNote database you want to use.

In the Figure 7.26, a reference has been inserted and a reference list generated. Additional references will be added automatically to this list, as you continue writing and inserting references.

You may want to change the output style of the reference list. To do this, choose a style from the 'Style' list on the EndNote tab (Figure 7.27). If the style

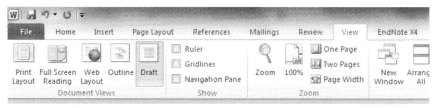

To insert a reference, click on 'Insert Citation'. Enter the search term and click on 'Find'. Then double click on the reference you want to insert. Good reference management is an important part of systematically reviewing the literature[1].

References

1. Torgerson C. *Systematic Reviews*: Continuum International Publishing Group, 2003.

Figure 7.26 A citation and reference inserted in a Word document using EndNote

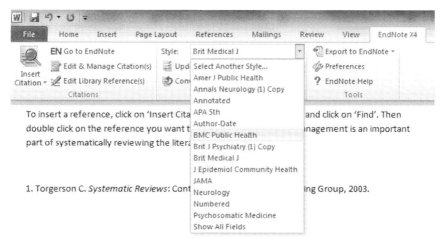

Figure 7.27 Choosing a bibliographic style in EndNote

you want is not shown, choose 'Select Another Style'. Additional styles can be downloaded from the EndNote website (http://endnote.com/downloads/styles).

Summary

This chapter has explained how to use the major search tools used in the health sciences in order to conduct your research, stay up to date, and inform your day-to-day work. The chapter has differentiated between narrative reviews and systematic reviews. Narrative reviews describe key studies in the field and provide a selective summary of your topic, and are therefore subject to bias and omissions. Systematic reviews provide a more thorough and comprehensive study of a topic, help you to find the most relevant publications, and provide a method which another researcher could replicate. To help you conduct this kind of literature search, the chapter has explained in detail how to design a systematic research strategy that will enable you to find, save and process the most relevant research in your field, using the useful PICO acronym to focus your research questions and using Boolean operators to refine your search terms. It has shown why you should search at least two databases to cross-reference your results and draw inclusively on multidisciplinary research and overlapping sources, and suggested some useful current databases as well as other less formal sources of research such as conferences and social media. It has stressed the importance of keeping good records throughout the process in order to manage the review and to allow others to replicate your research, and has also shown that a systematic review can be an effective piece of original research in its own right. It has also explained how to manage your research results, by exporting references from your search into CiteULike which allows you to swiftly store and organise your sources, process your results, and export references into bibliographic software such as EndNote or Reference Manager when you are writing up your research. Using a web-based citation library like CiteULike enables you to access your search results from anywhere, and share them with other users.

You should now feel confident to conduct narrative and systematic reviews, incorporate the results into your work, and design new research questions which will enable you to build on the existing research and make a contribution to your field. The next three chapters show you how to critically appraise the literature, enabling you to assess and evaluate the relevance and usefulness of published work to your particular research topic.

Web links

http://www.academia.edu
http://www.nlm.nih.gov/bsd/disted/pubmedtutorial/
http://www.youtube.com/watch?v=LkNeEUV4sPs
http://endnote.com/training
http://www.refman.com/training/
http://www.cochrane.org/training

## 8

Randomised controlled trials

This chapter presents three examples of how the critical appraisal approach can be applied to randomised controlled trials (RCTs). Each of the trials is quite different, but they share essentially the same study design. Extracts have been reproduced from each paper, and important parts of the papers are also shown, but you should read each paper in full if you want to get the most out of the chapter. All three are open access journal articles, meaning that you can obtain them free of charge.

The chapter will help you to critically evaluate questions (adapted from the Critical Appraisal Skills Programme (CASP) website [116]) such as:

- Does the study ask a clearly focused question?

- Was the question focused in terms of the population studied?

- Was the question focused in terms of the intervention studied?

- Was the question focused in terms of the outcomes considered?

- How appropriate were the research methods used?

- How were the research participants chosen and what might the composition of the participant groups tell us?

- How was the study followed up and how was data collected?

- How are the results presented and what is the main result?

- How precise are the results and how can we apply them in future?

Before proceeding it is useful to list the three trials discussed in this chapter:

- a cognitive behavioural intervention to reduce sexually transmitted infections among gay men: randomised trial;

- the effect on smoking quit rate of telling patients their lung age: the Step2quit randomised controlled trial;

- effect of physical activity on cognitive function in older adults at risk for Alzheimer's disease: a randomised trial.

As well as helping you to understand how randomised controlled trials work, the chapter is intended to help you think critically about the trials conducted by others, enabling you to evaluate the usefulness of published results of such trials to your work, and also setting out signposts which will enable you to design such trials yourself.

Intended learning outcomes

By the end of this chapter, you should be able to:

- identify the essential features of an RCT;
- read and understand published journal articles which report the results of RCTs;
- critically appraise a journal article or paper describing the results of an RCT;
- summarise the strengths and limitations of a paper describing an RCT.

Introducing key terms

Part of the difficulty of appraising an RCT or another type of study as a student, is that you may be unfamiliar with the topic, the research methods and statistics used in the study. If you don't understand what the authors of the paper did, how can you comment on the quality of the paper? It is worth noting however, that even if you don't understand all of the details of a study, a well-written paper should be understandable without having to know all these details. Even if you have no prior knowledge of the area, research papers are structured and presented in a way that should make them as accessible as possible. To illustrate, the three papers chosen for this chapter concern quite different topics.

Kinds of research questions

An RCT can address focused research questions that concern a population, intervention, control group and some outcome. Recall that the acronym PICO is helpful to remember when you try to identify the research question which an RCT was designed to address:

- *Participants*: What sample, and from what population?
- *Intervention*: What is the intervention, treatment or exposure?
- *Control*: Who are the control group? Were participants randomised?
- *Outcome:* What was the outcome? How was it measured?

What are the essential features of an RCT?

In the hierarchy of evidence, RCT designs are placed at the top. This is because RCTs can address both known and unknown confounding factors, because randomisation ensures that differences between treatment and control groups are minimised. Additionally, it is usually clear that the treatment or intervention is responsible for any difference in the outcome. In contrast, observational studies (e.g. cohort studies, Chapter 9) require researchers to adjust for known confounding factors in the analysis, and cannot address unknown confounders. There are three features of an RCT which should be distinguished:

1 *Randomisation*: Participants should have an equal probability of receiving a new intervention or being in the 'control' condition. This is achieved by randomisation. If successful, randomisation ensures that differences between the treatment and control groups are minimised. This addresses both known and unknown confounding factors, by distributing them randomly across both groups.

2 *A control group*: The control group does not receive the intervention which is of interest. They either receive treatment as usual, treatment according to existing guidelines or a placebo (e.g. a sugar pill). Participants and/or staff involved in the study may or may not be 'blinded', a term explained below:

   a *Single blinded*: If the RCT has been single blinded, participants do not know which group they are in (treatment or control).

   b *Double blinded:* In double blinded trials, neither participants nor research staff know which group participants were assigned to.

   c *Triple blinded*: In triple blinded trials, participants, research staff and data analysts do not know which group participants were assigned to.

3 *An intervention*: As indicated by the term 'trial', an RCT evaluates some intervention, procedure or drug. It is important to note that not all trials are randomised, controlled or blinded.

It is worth noting that the terms single, double and triple blinding have started to fall out of favour. Double and triple blinding can mean different

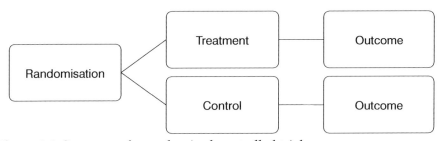

Figure 8.1 Structure of a randomised controlled trial

things to different people, causing ambiguity. The CONSORT statement recommends that researchers simply explain who was blinded, and how this was achieved [51]. If researchers follow this recommendation, then this should make it easier to understand whether an RCT involved blinding, and the impact this might have on how we interpret the results.

A cognitive behavioural intervention to reduce sexually transmitted infections among gay men: randomised trial [52]

We will appraise this first paper in more detail than the next two papers, because concepts will be introduced for the first time with which you may be unfamiliar. This paper attracted great interest when it was published back in 2001, because very few attempts had been made to evaluate whether cognitive behavioural therapy (CBT) could be used to reduce sexual risk-taking among gay/bisexual men. When this RCT was conducted, human immunodeficiency virus (HIV) infection rates had started to rise again and this has continued. HIV has high morbidity, mortality, treatment and care costs. Left untreated, it usually leads to acquired immune deficiency syndrome (AIDS), leading to severe damage to the immune system. Self-reported condom use is often found to be higher among gay/bisexual men than among heterosexuals [53]. This is attributed partly to the success of community-based interventions, such as peer education, and partly to an early response to the HIV epidemic during the 1980s [54]. However, men who have sex with men account for the largest proportion of new HIV infections acquired in the UK. For this reason, they are a priority for interventions to reduce HIV and other sexually transmitted infections (STIs).

> Download this paper from http://www.ncbi.nlm.nih.gov/pmc/articles/ PMC32307/

Did the study ask a clearly focused question?

We can find the research question towards the end of the introduction. It is not phrased as a research question explicitly, but the authors do tell us what they wanted to know and how they intended to find out:

> We developed a small group intervention aimed at gay men, which draws on several psychological models of behavioural change. We evaluated its effects in a pragmatic randomised controlled trial using clinical end points (new sexually acquired infections) as well as self-reported changes in behaviour (p. 1452).

Was the question focused in terms of the population studied?

The population is defined reasonably clearly, but we are not told how men were deemed to be 'homosexual'. Presumably this was based on self-reported sexual behaviour as being with men only, but the authors do not say how bisexual men were classified. The inconsistent terminology used throughout the manuscript adds to the ambiguity. The intervention was 'aimed at gay men' but not all men who have sex with men identify as 'gay', a frequently observed feature of some ethnic minority groups. In epidemiology, the term 'men who have sex with men' is used for precisely this reason – it clearly focuses the population in terms of their behaviour, rather than their identity, which is a different component of sexual orientation

Was the question focused in terms of the intervention studied?

The intervention is described briefly and we are referred to the *British Medical Journal* (*BMJ*) website for a more detailed description. Owing to restrictions on space, it is often difficult for authors to describe complex interventions in detail. Complex interventions can be compared to medicines that might have several active 'ingredients'. It is difficult to determine which part of the intervention might have an effect. The Medical Research Council (MRC) guidelines on complex interventions [55] were developed in order to improve the way in which complex interventions are conducted and reported. The intervention drew on 'several psychological models', adding to the complexity. Have a look at the description of the intervention, and see if you can determine exactly what the intervention involved. This is not easy. This kind of intervention has also been described as a 'black box' intervention, a metaphor referring to a process that cannot be observed directly in order to determine exactly what happened. The term 'pragmatic RCT' is often used in this kind of situation, where the intervention is less clearly defined.

Was the question focused in terms of the outcomes considered?

The outcomes considered are clearly described. Clinics and laboratory diagnoses were used to identify new STIs, and questionnaires were used to record self-reported behaviour change, which is an established and acceptable method. There is no practical alternative to self-reported sexual behaviour.

In summary, the research question was clearly focused on a population (gay/bisexual men), intervention (CBT), control group (treatment as usual) and outcome (STIs).

Overall, we can conclude that it is worth continuing to read this paper, because it is focused and is the right kind of study for the research question. Therefore, we move on to more detailed questions about the study.

Was this an RCT and was it appropriately so?

The study was an RCT, and this is appropriate for evaluating new interventions. Participants were randomised, discussed in more detail below. There was a control group.

Were participants appropriately allocated to intervention and control groups?

Participants were randomly allocated using sealed opaque envelopes. This is probably sufficient, but we need to be careful that baseline differences between the intervention and control groups do not exist. Particularly when sample sizes are small, randomisation can still result in intervention and control groups that differ in respect to one or more important variables. One method of addressing this is to first stratify participants (e.g. by age groups) and then randomise within each group. No method of balancing is reported, but we can look at the paper's Table 1 to determine if the groups were different after randomisation. This shows that the intervention group and control group were not significantly different, meaning that randomisation worked. There are two important differences between those who declined to participate and those who were randomly allocated into the study, however: education and ethnicity:

1 non-white people eligible for the study were more likely to decline to participate ($p = .06$, indicating a non-significant trend);

2 men with secondary school education or lower were significantly more likely to decline ($p = .04$).

These kinds of differences can be important, because this means that non-white and less educated men were under-represented in the study. It is also worth noting that men were randomised as individuals, but 18 had a long-term partner and were assigned to the same arm as their partner. This is not random, which the author addressed by removing these participants from the analysis. We cannot determine the impact of the intervention on couples, this being a different research question. There were also potentially important differences between those who attended the workshop intervention and those who completed the questionnaire at 12 months:

1 attenders were significantly more likely to have attended one before ($p = .01$);

2 attenders were more likely to complete the questionnaire at 12 months ($p < .001$);

3 those completing the questionnaire were significantly older ($p < .001$).

Were participants, staff and study personnel 'blind' to participants' study groups?

With an intervention that consists of a training course, it is obviously not possible to blind participants to the fact that they are in the intervention condition. The research staff analysing the data were blinded. Arguably, blinding does not matter in this study. We might worry about Hawthorne effects, even in the participants who did not receive the intervention but were asked to complete postal questionnaires. The emphasis on clinical end points, outcomes which study personnel were blind to, addresses these concerns to some extent.

Were all of the participants who entered the trial accounted for at its conclusion?

None of the intervention group participants got a control group option, which can sometimes happen in trials if patients cannot receive the intervention for some reason. The flow diagram reported in the paper does a good job of showing that all participants were accounted for. This is one reason why the CONSORT recommendations include a flow diagram – they are extremely helpful. It is worth noting that there was loss to follow-up and this appears to differ between the two groups. A total of 59 of the intervention group and 40 of the control group were lost to follow-up, but other than withdrawing from the study, emigration or death, there is a large category "other loss to follow-up" which is really twice as large in the intervention group (42 men in the intervention group, 24 in the control group).

Were all participants in all groups followed up and data collected in the same way?

The methods of data collection were the same in both groups. Participants in both conditions were followed up in the same way (questionnaires and clinical end points), although as mentioned above, we don't know why "other loss to follow-up" was twice as high in the intervention condition. Men in the control group however, did not receive the same amount of attention from researchers and health workers. A placebo effect induced by men taking part in the workshop can be addressed because the groups are randomised. Hawthorne effects however, may remain, because even men receiving questionnaires in the control group are receiving 'attention' from researchers or healthcare workers. Uptake of counselling and other prevention services was not significantly different between the two groups. We do not need to worry therefore, about men attending the workshop and then deciding to obtain counselling. If this had happened, we might worry that the counselling rather than the workshop had influenced the outcome.

Did the study have enough participants to minimise the play of chance?

A power calculation was reported, but only for the primary outcomes (see Appendix 6: Statistical Power). The authors wanted to detect a reduction in the number of newly acquired sexually transmitted infections from 20 per cent (the current incidence rate for one year) to 8 per cent, and a reduction in unprotected anal intercourse (UAI) from 50 per cent to 30 per cent. It is not clear why a reduction in UAI from 50 per cent to 30 per cent has been chosen. This is equivalent to using a condom with 5 out of 10 partners, compared to using a condom with 7 out of 10 partners. No distinction was made between regular and casual partners. To some extent, the effect size chosen is arbitrary, particularly for a new intervention because the effectiveness of the intervention is not known. If the intervention works, but has a smaller effect size, then the study may have required more participants in order to have the statistical power necessary to detect it. Loss to follow-up was estimated to be 25 per cent by the authors.

How are the results presented and what is the main result?

The main results are presented in Table 2 (UAI) and Table 3 (STIs). Let's look at the results from Table 2 first, which show the association between having the intervention and UAI reported in the past month. The numerator/denominators show the proportion reporting UAI out of the total, presumably the total without missing data because these numbers do not match the totals shown for each group (column headers).

In the paper, results are also shown for UAI in the past year and for partners with a different or unknown HIV status. The intervention and control groups are compared. There are no significant differences between them. We can see a trend towards the intervention reducing UAI at six months ($p = .07$) but this is not statistically significant at the traditional $p = .05$ level. This may be a small effect which was not detected because of low statistical power. The main result here is that the intervention did not significantly reduce UAI at six months or 12 months, adjusting for STIs and baseline UAI.

The odds ratio and 95 per cent confidence intervals for STIs are shown in Table 3, and these are the 'clinical endpoints' which the authors are keen to emphasise because of their objectivity. There is an association between receiving the intervention and all new infections, a broad definition covering hepatitis B, herpes, genital warts, syphilis, gonorrhoea, chlamydia and non-specific urethritis (NSU). The odds ratio is 1.69 (95% CI, 95% CI 1.03, 2.77) which would seem to indicate that the intervention has actually *increased* the risk of STIs in the year of follow-up! After adjustment for infections at recruitment however, this reduces to 1.66 (95% CI 1.00 to 2.74) which is not statistically significant

Table 8.1 Table 2 from 'A cognitive behavioural intervention to reduce sexually transmitted infections among gay men: randomised trial'

	Baseline		6 months		12 months	
	Interven-tion (n = 175)	*Control* (n = 168)	*Interven-tion* (n = 137)	*Control* (n = 139)	*Interven-tion* (n = 116)	*Control* (n = 128)
UAI in the past month	63/172	50/166	32/136	44/136	31/114	39/124
p value (adjusting for STIs at baseline and whether behaviour was reported at baseline)				p = .07		p = .31

because the confidence intervals include 1. For a more specific definition of STIs comprising 'bacterial infections' (syphilis, chlamydia, gonorrhoea), there was no association before or after adjustment, although the effect was in the direction of increasing risk (OR = 1.84 after adjustment). Possible reasons for this are discussed by the authors in their discussion section, and we will think about this later.

Results other than the main results are often described as 'secondary outcomes'. It is important to focus on primary outcomes because these were the original focus of the study, and the study was powered for the primary outcomes. Secondary outcomes are more likely to produce chance findings, because they involve making additional comparisons. However, secondary outcomes can often be informative and can help us understand some of the main findings. Here are some of them:

- no association between the intervention and use of other clinics or community prevention services (Table 3);

- improvement in several self-reported psychometric measures in the questionnaire at follow-up (Table 4)

  - an improvement in communication skills of 0.23 points (95% CI 0.02, 0.45);

  - an improvement in safer sex efficacy of 0.25 points (95% CI 0.03 to 0.47);

  - an improvement in interpersonal barriers of 0.28 points (95% CI 0.07, 0.49).

Since sexual risk-taking might be reduced by some of these psychological mechanisms, it might be worth noting that the intervention had some effect on these. However, these could have arisen by chance and the study was not powered to detect changes on these secondary outcomes. These are not the true end points for the study, and it is not wise to consider them as surrogate endpoints – we cannot simply assume that these differences would eventually translate into a reduction in STIs at a later stage.

How precise are the results?

The confidence intervals for the results are quite wide, which may reflect the modest sample size. For UAI, no confidence intervals are reported (Table 2) although a *p* value is reported (see above). Concerning new STIs, the lower end of the interval is 1.03 and the upper end is 2.77. If you had to decide whether or not to implement this intervention, your decision might not be the same at the lower end as the upper end. After adjusting for baseline STIs, the lower end of the interval is 1.00 (no difference) and the upper end is 2.74 (around 2.7 times more likely to acquire new STIs). Leaving aside the problem that the direction of the effect seems to go in the wrong direction, the estimated effect is not precise.

Were all important outcomes considered so the results can be applied?

The decision about whether results from a paper should be applied will depend on your situation, and on many other factors. Rarely will a single paper lead to a new intervention being adopted. For the purpose of the current paper, let's assume that you are a public health consultant and are unsure whether or not to provide funding for this intervention in your local area. Will the workshop reduce STIs among gay/bisexual men? Here are some issues we should consider:

1 The people included in the trial could be different from the local population. Men attending clinics may be more health aware, may have engaged in more UAI, may have more casual partners, and may have different socio-economic characteristics. White and more educated men were over-represented in the study. Some men were lost from the intervention group and we cannot determine why.

2 Did loss to follow-up in the intervention group reflect low acceptability of the intervention? Did some participants react negatively to the workshop? Very little information is provided. Indeed, the intervention was originally designed to be three separate workshops, but was shortened because too few men attended all of them.

3 The local setting may differ from that of the trial, which was London based. Gay/bisexual men are a 'hard to reach' population and STI clinics do not provide a representative sample of this population. This may not be the best place to recruit such men for an intervention of this kind, particularly if we wanted to target MSM (men who have sex with men) who do not identify as gay/bisexual.

4 We may not be able to provide the same intervention. Although some information is provided about the intervention on the BMJ website, complex interventions are difficult to replicate [55]. The exact content of the workshop is not known, and the delivery method may change if we tried to replicate it. There are aspects of the intervention which are difficult to measure (e.g. rapport between the trainer and the participants, levels of trust, enjoyment during the day). Would it matter to the participants if the trainer identified as gay/bisexual, or male/female, for example?

5 The primary outcomes were not significantly changed, although a trend toward UAI reducing was apparent. There was a slightly worrying trend towards an *increase* in STIs following the intervention. We should be careful about unintended consequences, which the authors suggest may have occurred if attendees moved from UAI to other kinds of sexual activities, such as oral sex. It would be useful to look at each STI separately in a larger study – is the reduction in UAI likely to translate into fewer HIV infections, but more STIs of other kinds, and does the cost/benefit of this situation matter? HIV is more expensive to treat than STIs, many of which are fully treatable. The benefit to individuals

(improved communication, safer sex efficacy and interpersonal barriers) may need to be balanced with a potential increase in STIs, which would not benefit the wider population. These are two competing perspectives. Policy makers may also have to consider the cost of treating additional STIs. The study may need to be replicated with a larger sample, in order to determine if and why this unintended effect actually occurs.

6 Policy and practice should not change as a result of the evidence contained in this trial, without further research. It may have unintended consequences, and we do not know enough about the intervention in order to implement it (or to rule it out altogether). An intervention that has efficacy during a trial may not have effectiveness when it is introduced in practice, and low acceptability is one of many reasons why interventions that work in trials do not always work in practice.

The discussion section contains a summary of the main findings, the strengths and weaknesses (according to the authors – it is important to appraise your own perceived strengths and weaknesses as you read it), comparison to other studies, meaning of the study and possible implications. The authors suggest that 'the intervention was more likely to be harmful' but remember that this was not significant after adjustment. There is a suggestion that the intervention discouraged UAI but encouraged 'low risk, non-penetrative sex', although this effect attenuated over time leading the authors to describe this as a 'transient' effect. The authors correctly note that the broad and narrow definitions of sexual behaviour may have masked the true situation. It would have been interesting to see HIV versus other STIs and a cost-effectiveness calculation, although these are usually not reported in the same paper as the main results from an RCT. You may not agree that self-reported outcomes 'tend to overestimate benefits', particularly when these outcomes can only be evaluated using self-report (e.g. condom use, self-efficacy, communication). Also, the study was not powered to detect changes in all of these secondary outcomes. The study focused on clinical end points but other end points matter to different people – the participants themselves, for example, might view a reduction in UAI but an increased risk of STIs other than HIV as acceptable. Clinicians may have different views.

In conclusion, the paper reports a generally well-designed RCT but raises several new questions:

1 How many sessions are necessary, and it is necessary to reduce the intervention from three to one sessions?

2 Is the workshop acceptable to gay/bisexual men and more generally, to MSM? How can it be replicated and standardised? Which aspect of the workshop is most successful?

3 If the workshop results in reduced UAI but a transient increase in risk of STIs because lower risk behaviour is adopted instead, is the additional risk worth the reduction in risk from new HIV infections? A cost-effectiveness analysis would be helpful here.

4 What do the men prioritise themselves, reducing new HIV infections or reducing all infections considered equally harmful? It is unlikely that all STIs have equal salience/importance for this group.

5 Does the author's own view that such interventions can have the 'unintended effect of encouraging greater sexual activity' introduce a political dimension into the research? The authors have previously suggested that promoting condom use could increase sexual risk-taking [56] and that 'it is hard to show that condom promotion has had any effect on HIV epidemics'. Such views are controversial. The 'partner reduction' approach has been used to claim that people should 'abstain' from casual sexual encounters, which LGBT community activists have objected to on ethical and political grounds.

6 We should also consider the politics of HIV prevention funding at the time as the study was conducted. Clinical services were often competing with community organisations in order to obtain funding to deliver HIV prevention interventions. Many gay men's health organisations used peer education approaches, and some used CBT. It was difficult to show that peer education had an influence on HIV transmission. Evidence that CBT has an impact on STIs or on sexual behaviour could have been used to argue for a change in how funding was allocated. This could disadvantage community interventions, who would find it more difficult to collect evidence on how their approaches might influence these outcomes.

Effect on smoking quit rate of telling patients their lung age: the Step2quit randomised controlled trial [57]

Practitioners working in several disciplines in the health sciences, particularly public health and primary care, are always keen to identify ways to encourage people to stop smoking. This research into the effect of telling patients their 'lung age' on subsequent quitting is therefore quite interesting. Biomarkers have been used in other settings as tools to motivate patients to change behaviour, but a Cochrane Review found few studies that had used RCT designs [58]. Lung function offers a relatively cheap, and therefore potentially cost-effective, way to motivate patients to quit smoking. Telling patients their lung age is a psychological technique designed to motivate this behaviour change.

Download this paper from http://www.bmj.com/content/336/7644/598

Did the study ask a clearly focused question?

Was the question focused in terms of the population studied?

The authors are very clear about the population they have studied. Their introduction explains that chronic obstructive pulmonary disease (COPD) can be detected as young as age 35, but on average it is detected at age 50. Focusing the study on smokers at age 35 or older is therefore sensible, because we need to know more about how to encourage quitting earlier in midlife:

> We searched computerised patient records from five general practices in Hertfordshire to identify people aged 35 and over who had been recorded as a smoker in the previous 12 months (p.2).

There were several exclusion criteria, most of them to ensure that people with pre-existing disease were not included. This focuses the population on smokers without disease at baseline.

Was the question focused in terms of the intervention studied?

The intervention is focused and described clearly. Figures 1 and 2 in the paper illustrate how patients were shown their 'lung age'. The paragraph 'Information given to participants' provides sufficient information for this trial to be replicated, because anyone reading the paper could find out what the intervention involved.

Was the question focused in terms of the outcomes considered?

The primary outcome was smoking cessation at 12 months, confirmed by salivary cotinine testing. Secondary outcomes were less focused, but included the number of cigarettes smoked and newly diagnosed COPD. There are two other outcomes reported in Table 3 which are not covered in detail in the paper (attended NHS smoking clinics, used smoking cessation help).

In summary, the research question was clearly focused on a population (adults aged 35 or older), intervention (telling patients their lung age), control group (treatment as usual) and outcome (smoking cessation).

Was this an RCT and was it appropriately so?

The study was an RCT, appropriate for evaluating the effectiveness of interventions. Participants were randomised, and there was a control group who received usual care.

Were participants appropriately allocated to intervention and control groups?

Participants were randomly allocated using sealed opaque envelopes, which contained a computer generated number (odd numbered envelopes received the intervention). Table 2 shows the baseline characteristics of the intervention and control groups. It does not however, show results from statistical tests that can help determine if the groups were significantly different at baseline or not. In the text, we are informed that the control group contained 'significantly more people with a history of stroke' (p.4) and that there were 'few differences', but it would have been nice to see p values in Table 2 for all variables. Baseline differences can occur by chance, even after randomisation, so the higher rate of stroke in the control group is not a major cause for concern.

Were participants, staff and study personnel 'blind' to participants' study groups?

The clerk who dealt with randomisation using sealed envelopes took no further part in the study. Although it is highly unlikely that the study team would try to influence which patients received the intervention, it is theoretically possible, so this statement was probably included simply to reassure those readers who are particularly sceptical. The staff administering the intervention clearly knew that they were giving the intervention, because they were telling patients their lung age. This is a necessary limitation of the study design because blinding is not feasible here.

Were all of the participants who entered the trial accounted for at its conclusion?

The flow diagram in Figure 3 shows that the authors have followed the CONSORT guidelines, showing what happened to participants throughout the trial. Loss to follow-up was fairly low, around 11 per cent in both groups, much lower than the 50 per cent which the study team expected. It is not clear why 50 per cent was expected, but the low rate of loss to follow-up could indicate characteristics of the sample which are associated with greater participation in health research, such as higher socio-economic status (SES), health consciousness or interest in the study. It is quite unusual to have such a high participation rate after one year.

Were all participants in all groups followed up and data collected in the same way?

All participants in both groups were followed up and data collected in the same way, for the primary outcome measure. There were some differences in how the control group were treated, which existed by necessity. The control group were not given their lung age results but were invited to have a second test after 12 months (after the trial had finished) 'to see if there had been any change in lung function'. There was an option to 'receive a letter with more information from the research doctor within four weeks'. We are not told how many patients were sent this letter, and whether it contained standard spirometry results (simple FEV_1), lung age, or something else. If it contained lung age, this means that these participants in the control group actually received the intervention, which could be problematic. It might distort the results by underestimating the true effect of the intervention. The option to have a second test after 12 months, or a letter after 4 weeks, helps satisfy ethical guidelines that discourage researchers from withholding potentially helpful interventions or drugs. For trials that show beneficial effects of the intervention, it is arguably not ethical to withhold this intervention from the control group indefinitely. Some trials have been terminated early for similar reasons. For example, once it was established that aspirin was effective at reducing heart attack risk, the control group were given the intervention option. Ethical issues are discussed in Chapter 11 in more detail.

Did the study have enough participants to minimise the play of chance?

A statistical power calculation is reported, showing that 300 participants would produce 80 per cent power to detect an effect size of 10 per cent reduction in smoking cessation rate. The study team estimated an attrition rate of 50 per cent, although it is not clear where this figure comes from. Previous studies or pilot studies can be used to estimate attrition rates, or they can be simple guesstimates. Based on these figures, they aimed to recruit 600 participants. They achieved a sample size of 561, showing that the study was powered to detect a 10 per cent reduction, because this is greater than the 300 needed. The study was not powered to detect differences in secondary outcomes (daily cigarette consumption), or the two additional outcomes shown in Table 3 (attending smoking clinics, using cessation help).

How are the results presented and what is the main result?

The results are presented by comparing the number and percentage of participants in each group, who were confirmed as having quit smoking 12 months later (Table 3). In the control group, 18 (6.4 per cent) had quit. In the intervention group, 38 (13.6 per cent) had quit. The difference is 7.2 per cent, meaning that around 7 per cent more participants told their 'lung age' had quit, compared to those who were not told their lung age. The effect size is slightly smaller than the 10 per cent expected by the study team, but the sample size has still achieved sufficient statistical power to detect that this difference is statistically significant ($p = .01$). The p value indicates that it is highly unlikely that this difference is due to chance. It is worth noting that the actual lung age did not seem to matter, which is perhaps surprising.

How precise are the results?

The confidence intervals surrounding the difference of 7.2 per cent are shown (p.4) as 2.2 percent to 12.1 per cent. Although fairly wide, they do not include zero. We can be fairly sure that the effect is to increase, rather than decrease, smoking cessation. Even at the lower end of this interval (2.2 per cent), we would still conclude that the intervention encouraged people to quit smoking.

Were all important outcomes considered so the results can be applied?

As discussed above, other important outcomes were considered in the trial. Not only did the intervention improve the smoking cessation rate, it reduced the number of cigarettes smoked per day (Table 3). People in the intervention group smoked on average two cigarettes less (11.7 vs. 13.7 cigarettes) per day, 12 months later, compared to the control group. Although small, this effect was statistically significant ($p = .03$) and we need to keep in mind that small effects can be important when applied at the population level, and over time. The effect of larger populations of smokers reducing their consumption by two cigarettes per day, over many years, may have some benefit. The difference in the number of people attending NHS smoking clinics was not tested, presumably because of small numbers (5 vs. 4). The difference in those accessing cessation help was not significant ($p = .20$) but the study was not powered to detect this difference. Overall, we do not know what the effect of telling patients their lung age might be on outcomes other than quitting and cigarette reduction, but it is likely to be a beneficial effect.

The people in the trial could be different from your local population. Consider the setting. The characteristics of the Hertfordshire GP practices are not known, and we may want to consider the socio-economic profile of this region before making strong conclusions about the effectiveness of the intervention across the UK. Randomisation however, ensures that known and unknown confounding factors are addressed. If the intervention works, this is still good-quality evidence, but the evidence can only generalise to patients with a similar socio-economic profile. You can check the socio-economic profile of a region on the Network of Public Health Observatories website (www.apho.org.uk/default. aspx?RID=49802) under Health Profiles. In 2011 for example, Hertfordshire performed well on nearly all indicators of socio-economic status and health inequalities, with the exception of physical activity in children. Would this intervention be equally as effective in a region with high levels of deprivation and low levels of educational attainment, such as Wakefield (identified as an NHS 'Spearhead' region, performing poorly on many indicators)?

Finally, according to the stage of change theory cited in the paper, participants will move from a pre-contemplative stage, to contemplative, preparation and action stages, before quitting. Table 2 indicates that only around 20 per cent of participants were at the action stage in both conditions. If however, telling patients their lung age motivates them to take action, why hadn't more patients moved through these stages? There may be other mechanisms at work which the theory has not accounted for. As the authors note, the mechanism accounting for why this intervention works remains unknown. For now, our conclusion is that whatever the mechanism, it seems to work.

Effect of physical activity on cognitive function in older adults at risk for Alzheimer's disease: a randomised trial [59]

Many older adults do not meet the recommended levels of physical activity, which are published by the World Health Organisation [60]. Physical inactivity may be a risk factor for cognitive decline, mild cognitive impairment, and dementia [61]. Therefore, researchers have speculated whether physical activity may be a possible intervention, to slow down cognitive decline. The paper we will now critically appraise involved a physical activity intervention and its effects on cognitive decline over 18 months. Given that cognitive decline occurs over several decades [62], do keep in mind that this is a relatively short follow-up period, and we should therefore expect a small effect.

Download this paper from http://jama.jamanetwork.com/ article.aspx?articleid=182502

Did the study ask a clearly focused question?

Yes, the research question is stated at the end of the introduction section and it is clearly focused:

> We designed the present randomised trial to test whether a 24-week home-based physical activity intervention reduces the rate of cognitive decline among older adults at increased risk of dementia.

The population is defined as 'older adults…at increased risk of dementia', the intervention is 'a 24-week home-based physical activity intervention', there is presumably a control group (although we will have to check the methods section to be sure), and the outcome is 'the rate of cognitive decline' which presumably the authors predict will be slower in the intervention group at the end of follow-up. Therefore, all four of the PICO criteria have been described.

The control group and the intervention group both received standard materials covering memory loss, stress management, diet, alcohol and smoking but not physical activity. The intervention involved encouraging participants to perform 150 minutes of moderate intensity physical activity per week, in three 50-minute sessions. If already doing this at baseline, participants were asked to add another 50 minutes per week (one session). This was delivered as part of a one hour interview with a study team member and consisted of a home-based workbook, a diary that was mailed to the study team every month, and recommended activities such as walking (although participants were free to choose their activities). Eight newsletters were mailed out during the study, aimed at reinforcing the recommendations, which should also be considered part of the intervention.

In summary, the research question was clearly focused on a population (older adults at risk of dementia), intervention (physical activity), control group (treatment as usual) and outcome (cognitive decline).

Was this a randomised controlled trial (RCT) and was it appropriately so?

This was an RCT, which is the right research approach for evaluating the effectiveness of a new intervention. Since the population is studied in community settings, it may also provide useful information about the efficacy of the intervention.

Were participants appropriately allocated to intervention and control groups?

The 'Participants' section of the paper is rather complex, because there are several different inclusion criteria – even before we get to randomisation. Although the population was defined broadly as 'older adults', this section is more specific about the inclusion criteria:

- age 50 or older;

- attending memory clinics or responding to media advertisements;

- Telephone Interview for Cognitive Status (TICS) score of 19 or higher;

- Geriatric Depression Scale lower than 6;

- drinking 4 units of alcohol per day or less;

- no chronic mental illness (e.g. schizophrenia);

- no medical conditions likely to compromise survival (e.g cancer) or prevent engagement in physical activity (e.g. cardiac failure);

- no severe sensory impairment;

- fluent in written or spoken English.

On top of all these requirements, participants were then invited to a screening interview and were excluded if any of the following criteria were met:

- Mini-Mental State Examination score <24;

- Clinical Dementia Rating Scale score of 1 or more;

- unable to walk for six minutes without assistance.

Importantly, volunteers were eligible for randomisation if they answered yes to 'Do you have any difficulty with your memory?', regardless of whether or not any of the tests given showed an impairment. This means that participants had to report subjective memory complaints, which may not be reliable indicators of objective memory problems. Subjective complaints are often not associated with objective cognitive function, and may be confounded by depression and personality traits (particularly neuroticism or negative emotionality) [63]. This means that participants in the sample may be self-selected, to some extent, and the results may not generalise to patients who have memory problems but are not aware of them.

Mild cognitive impairment (MCI) was defined as having scores 1.5 SD lower than the age and sex-specific mean on four subtests (verbal fluency, object picture naming, word list immediate and delayed recall, praxis) from a battery of cognitive tests called the Cognitive Battery of the Consortium to Establish a Registry for Alzheimer's Disease. A reference is provided for this battery, should we want to find out more about it. It provides population norms, normative data, so that the study sample can be compared to the population. The 'Randomisation' section explains how eligible participants (after all of the above inclusion and exclusion criteria were met) were randomised. Randomisation was performed using computer generated numbers. Table 1 shows the baseline characteristics in each group, allowing us to check if randomisation worked. The groups look very similar, but there is no clear statement that these values were compared formally, to see if there were any statistically significant differences.

Were participants, staff and study personnel 'blind' to participants' study group?

The authors acknowledge that blinding was not really practical for this kind of intervention: 'Due to the nature of the intervention, participants were not blinded to group membership, but research personnel undertaking cognitive assessments were' (p. 1029). Additionally, participants were asked not to discuss the intervention with study staff. We should bear in mind that some participants might have done this anyway, which could potentially have introduced some bias. This risk was minimised by having analysis staff in a separate building from where the participants were seen.

Were all of the participants who entered the trial accounted for at its conclusion?

The authors provide a flow diagram (p. 1030 in the paper) which is helpful because it shows that all of the participants were accounted for, from recruitment to end of follow-up. Flow diagrams are recommended by the CONSORT statement [51]. We can see what happened to each participant, and who was lost. The figure shows that 85 people were in each condition (exercise and control), but that only 69 of these people came to the 18-month visit (6-, 12-, and 18-month follow-ups were performed). The reason why 85, rather than 69, people were included in the primary analysis is because they were analysed on an intention-to-treat basis. Multiple imputation was used to replace missing values, which often reduces bias compared to simply excluding participants with missing data from the analysis. The authors also conducted a complete-case analysis (repeating the results using only participants with complete data at all time points), allowing them to compare results and see if multiple imputation changed conclusions drawn. The information provided is detailed and reassuring.

Were the participants in all groups followed up and data collected in the same way?

Yes, both groups were followed up and data collected in the same way. This is clear from the flow diagram and from other results reported. It is worth noting however, that adherence to the recommended increase in physical activity in the intervention group was evaluated by using self-reported physical activity questionnaires. Self-reported physical activity may be under- or over-reported, introducing bias. It is also worth noting that according to this criterion, 78 per cent achieved adherence, meaning that 22 per cent did not actually receive the intervention as intended. Compare this to a drug trial, where not all participants in the drug condition actually take the drug as instructed – it could weaken any apparent effects.

Did the study have enough participants to minimise the play of chance?

A power calculation is reported (p. 1030). The effect size was estimated based on clinically meaningful differences of 2.5 points on the ADAS-cog, a cognitive test used to evaluate treatment effects in trials. To be able to detect an intervention effect capable of preventing a 2.5 point drop in cognitive function, a sample size of 168 was deemed necessary (85 in each group, drop-out estimated at 20 per cent, 90 per cent power). Since the sample size was 170, the study has adequate power to detect 2.5 point differences on ADAS-cog.

How are the results presented and what is the main result?

The bottom line results are that the exercise group experienced significantly less cognitive decline than the control group (see Table 2 in the paper, p.1032). At 18 months for example, the exercise group had ADAS-cog scores −0.38 lower than their baseline score, and the control group had scores 0.45 higher. Overall (across 6, 12 and 18 months), this was statistically ($p = .04$) but not clinically significant (given the definition of 2.5 points as clinically significant). The authors acknowledge this small effect: 'The average improvement of 0.69 points on the ADAS-Cog score compared with the usual care control group at 18 months is small but potentially important when one considers the relatively modest amount of physical activity undertaken by participants in the study'. The study was not powered to examine decline on other cognitive tests, although a significant result was found for word lists. This could be due to chance.

How precise are the results?

The precision of the results is difficult to gauge because of the way in which the results in Table 2 are presented. The confidence intervals shown refer to the mean difference from baseline in each group. It might have been more informative to see the mean difference between groups and the confidence intervals surrounding this mean difference. A figure might have been more useful. Nonetheless, the p value of .04 indicates that the intervention group had significantly better cognitive function compared to the control group.

Were all important outcomes considered so the results can be applied?

Adverse events were reported but were not thought to be caused by the intervention. Other points we might want to bear in mind, should we consider replicating this intervention in local settings, are that women were more likely to drop out than men. Secondary outcomes might include performance on specific tests, other than general ADAS-cog score, in a larger study with more statistical power, in future. In the complete case analysis (Table 4 in the paper, p. 1034), there is a non-significant trend suggesting better Mental Component Summary (MCS) scores in the intervention group (p = .08). Although the study was not powered to detect this effect, it is suggestive that the intervention might also have secondary benefits, including improved mental health, worth exploring in other studies. We should also note, as acknowledged by the authors, that the sample was relatively young and healthy, were drawn from a single community, mechanisms that might explain the effect are not known, the study was not designed to evaluate subsequent dementia risk, and not all participants received the intervention as intended, because they did not do the recommended levels of exercise. Additionally, only participants with subjective memory complaints were eligible, excluding those with objective but perhaps unrecognised complaints. Overall, the study was well-executed but a cost-effectiveness calculation would be required, given the small effect which the intervention produced. Is the cost of the intervention worth the small improvement in ADAS-cog scores?

Summary

In this chapter, we have performed a critical appraisal of three randomised controlled trials: a cognitive behavioural intervention for gay/bisexual men aimed at reducing sexually transmitted infections, telling patients their lung age and its effect on quitting smoking 12 months later, and a physical activity intervention for older adults and its effect on cognitive decline over 18 months. All three studies were selected because they provided you with experience in appraising quite different kinds of populations, interventions and outcome measures. All three share important characteristics: they involved randomisation, they had controlled groups, and they were trials. The most important thing to remember about RCTs is that they deal with both known and unknown confounding factors, which can produce good-quality evidence.

## 9

Cohort studies

This chapter presents three examples of how to critically appraise cohort studies. A cohort is a group of people who share common characteristics or experiences; for example, they were born within a particular period (a birth cohort); they may have been exposed to a particular risk factor for disease; or they may have undergone a particular medical procedure. A cohort study is a form of research design which longitudinally observes a group of people with particular attributes in order to monitor the health outcomes, for example, a cohort exposed to cigarette smoke in order to discover how many of them develop cancer. A cohort study can be conducted either prospectively, or retrospectively (historically) from existing recorded data.

The critical issues you will engage with are similar to those discussed in the previous chapter:

- Did the study address a clearly focused issue?

- Did the study use an appropriate method to answer the research question?

- Was the cohort recruited in an acceptable way?

- Was exposure (to risk), and study outcome, accurately measured to minimise bias?

- Have the authors identified all the important confounding factors, including those which are part of the design and analysis?

- Was follow up of subjects complete enough and long enough?

- What are the results of the study, and how precise are they?

- Do you believe the results, important for a cohort study, which may involve self-reporting? Can the results be applied to the local population, and do they fit with the other available evidence?

The studies discussed in this chapter are:

- environmental tobacco smoke and tobacco related mortality in a prospective study of Californians, 1960–98;

- joint effect of cigarette smoking and alcohol consumption on mortality;
- institutional risk factors for norovirus outbreaks in Hong Kong elderly homes: a retrospective cohort study.

Intended learning outcomes

By the end of this chapter, you should be able to:

- identify the essential features of a cohort study;
- read and understand published journal articles which report the results of cohort studies;
- critically appraise a journal article or paper describing the results of a cohort study;
- summarise the strengths and limitations of a paper describing a cohort study.

What are the essential features of a cohort study?

Cohort studies generally fall into one of two types:

- *Prospective cohort study*: the researchers identify whether or not participants have been exposed to a risk/protective factors, then follow-up the participants to see what happens to them. The disease outcome is not known at the start of the study. Did the participants get the disease or not?
- *Retrospective cohort study*: The disease outcome is known at the start of the study. The researchers then identify whether or not participants were exposed to the risk/protective factor in their past.

Prospective cohort studies are generally more common than retrospective cohort studies. In this chapter, we will appraise two prospective cohort studies and one retrospective one. Retrospective studies may rely on self-reported exposures by participants. For example, mothers may be asked how much coffee they drank during pregnancy. Patients attending a sexual health clinic may be asked how much alcohol they drank prior to their last sexual encounter. People attending a memory clinic may be asked about their usage of mobile phones in the years previously.

A clear limitation of retrospective studies is that the exposure status may not be accurate, due to recall bias. This could lead us to underestimate the association because misclassification will push the association towards a null effect. Stronger designs will obtain information about exposure status from other sources (e.g. record linkage to other databases). A limitation of prospective cohort studies is that researchers may have to wait a long time before finding out whether or not participants develop the disease outcome. It may be quicker to go for the retrospective approach, starting with a group of people who may or may not already have the disease. A case-control design (Chapter 10) is another possibility, particularly if the disease is rare.

Environmental tobacco smoke and tobacco related mortality in a prospective study of Californians, 1960–98 [64]

This paper generated much debate when it was published. The debates centred around the role of the tobacco industry which contributed some of the funding. Perhaps unfairly, many of the responses and letters about the paper did not appraise the results themselves. It is the methods, data, and analysis of a study which we should focus on, not the funding source. It is helpful however, to know a little of the background/context to this paper. The authors are known for their claims that the harms associated with environmental exposure may have been exaggerated by public health staff and policy makers, and have called for balanced appraisal of the harms and benefits of smoking bans.

Download this paper from http://www.bmj.com/content/326/7398/1057

Did the study address a clearly focused issue?

The study addresses a clearly focused issue, in terms of the population, risk factor(s), the outcome and whether they tried to detect a harmful or beneficial effect:

- The population is adults in California who originally took part in a study of cancer prevention in 1959 ($N = 1,078,894$) and who were followed until 1998. They were age 30–96 at baseline.

- The risk factor is exposure to second-hand smoke (environmental tobacco smoke), with particular reference to the 'never' smokers who had a smoking spouse.

- The outcome is tobacco related mortality, which includes deaths from coronary heart disease (CHD), lung cancer, chronic obstructive pulmonary disease (COPD) related to smoking in spouses.

- The effect is hypothesised to be harmful, although the authors are keen to emphasise that several studies and meta-analyses have not found a reliable association between environmental tobacco smoke and mortality.

Did the authors use an appropriate method to answer their question?

A cohort study is a good way of answering the question under the circumstances. It would not be ethical or feasible to expose people to second-hand smoke in a randomised controlled trial, for example. Animal experiments would be an alternative, but ethics committees (see Chapter 11) may question whether other kinds of evidence can be looked at first, before considering animal work. Additionally, animal studies may lack external validity (see Appendix 7), because the research question is concerned with the domestic second-hand smoke which the partners and children of smokers are exposed to in domestic settings.

Was the cohort recruited in an acceptable way?

Many papers that describe results from cohort studies do not include details about recruitment, because they can provide a reference to an earlier paper which provides those details. It would be unfeasible for a large cohort study to describe details of recruitment each time a paper was published. Cohort studies are usually expensive, involve many exposure variables, and several outcomes. Many papers are published from the same study, focusing on one research question at a time. Sensibly, the authors provide references to earlier papers which describe recruitment in more detail. Unfortunately this means that we would have to read these additional papers to learn more about recruitment. Here, the authors provide an earlier reference which describes the Cancer Prevention Study I cohort recruitment and follow-up in more detail [65, 66].

When appraising results from cohort studies, you may want to familiarise yourself with the cohort study itself. Although this involves extra reading, it can be helpful to learn about these cohorts. The *International Journal of Epidemiology* regularly publishes 'cohort profiles' which summarise major cohort studies, a helpful resource. Keep in mind that few cohorts are representative of the population, each share some common characteristic (e.g. birth years, time, place), and many are 'convenience cohorts'. This doesn't necessarily mean that results are biased, however, and often the evidence these cohorts produce is the best available evidence. We discuss issues of bias, external validity and generalisability in this and other chapters.

Was the exposure accurately measured to minimise bias?

The exposure was not measured objectively. Methods do exist for objective measurement of smoking, including passive smoking, such as salivary cotinine. This may not have been practical in this study, as in many studies, due to cost and the large sample size. This is not necessarily a serious limitation, but remember that misclassification of an exposure (e.g. some of the unexposed were actually exposed to the risk factor) can attenuate the association and push the OR towards 1 (no association). Relying on self-reported exposure can lead us to underestimate the effect of the exposure.

The participants are male never smokers, classified according to smoking status of their partner. The exposure was measured in male never smokers, the focus for analysis, and was classified 'according to the smoking status of the spouse: 1–9, 10–19, 20, 21–39, >=40 cigarettes per day' for men and women, with the addition of a pipe/cigar category for women. The reasons for these cut points, and the different approach to classifying pipe/cigar use for women is not clear, but may reflect peaks in the distribution at 10 and 20 cigarettes per day, and the fact that pipe/cigar use in women is relatively unusual.

To summarise, the exposure is "never smoker, married to current/ex-smoker" compared to "never smoker, married to never smokers". This ensures a 'clean' sample where the only smoking, in theory, is done by the spouse – not the study participant. This means that the exposure is environmental/passive smoking rather than primary smoking.

Was the outcome accurately measured to minimise bias?

Mortality is an objective outcome. The authors did not consider all-cause mortality but decided to focus on mortality related to CHD, lung cancer and COPD. It is unclear why they did not consider the broader category of cardiovascular disease deaths (CVD) in addition to the narrower category of CHD. CVD includes stroke deaths, for example, which CHD does not. Mortality records were obtained by matching participants on the California death file and the social security death index, to names, drivers' licences, dates of birth and heights. Some participants were not matched (p.4), which could lead to misclassification (e.g. classifying someone as alive who was actually dead).

Have the authors identified all important confounding factors?

The authors list seven confounding factors, in addition to age, which they think could be causally related both to the exposure (smoking status of the spouse) and the outcome (mortality): ethnic group, educational level, physical activity, body mass index, urbanisation (grouped into five population sizes), fruit/fruit juice intake and health status (good, fair, poor, sick). Additionally, analyses were repeated on all participants, then on those without baseline chronic diseases (cancer, heart disease, stroke). What other confounding factors do you think they might have missed? Socio-economic status is one possibility, which could be measured using occupation, income, or an area-based measure of socio-economic deprivation. We should also keep in mind that cohort studies can produce healthy survivor effects, meaning that healthier participants are more likely to remain in a study. This should be distinguished from 'health selection'.

Have they taken account of the confounding factors in the design and analysis?

The authors used Cox proportional hazards regression, so that they could adjust the relative risk of death over folow-up (hazard ratio) for the confounding factors listed above. We will learn more about adjustment in Chapters 13 and 14. They also conducted some sensitivity analyses, which involve repeating analyses to check whether the results were the same in those without baseline prevalent disease.

Was the follow up of subjects complete enough?

The cause of death was available for 93 per cent of the 79,437 deaths which were available for analysis. This is fairly complete. It is worth noting however, that deaths are sometimes classified into their primary 'underlying cause' and secondary causes. We assume here that this cause of death is the underlying cause, but environmental exposure to tobacco smoke might have influenced secondary causes of death. Completeness of follow-up is shown in detail in Table 1 in the paper. In 1999, another questionnaire was sent out to help clarify whether the matching process had been successful. This questionnaire showed that at least 99 per cent of the participants had been accurately matched.

Was the follow up of subjects long enough?

The analysis is based on three follow-ups (1959 = baseline/recruitment, 1965, and 1972; p.4) where the smoking status of the spouse was available. This is helpful because repeated assessments reduce measurement error in the exposure. If the authors had relied on smoking status of the spouse at baseline only, they would have missed possible changes in this status over time. The spouse might have stopped smoking or starting smoking, during follow-up, for example. The start time was set at 1960 (for convenience, the remainder of 1959 was excluded and so were 36 people who died in 1959 itself), until people had died, withdrawn from the study (defined as 'date last known alive'), or end of follow-up for the study (end of December 1998). Overall, 38 years of follow-up are available (1998–1960=38) which is sufficient time for deaths to occur. Because many participants will still be alive at follow-up, they have to be 'censored' from the analysis, which is why the authors chose Cox regression as a statistical model. Cox regression is beyond the scope of this introductory text, but it is worth noting here that Cox regression is appropriate because it takes into account this 'censoring' and deals only with the deaths that actually occurred during follow-up. Longer follow-up times result in more deaths, which results in more statistical power, because the regression model has more power if there are more deaths to consider. One of the most famous studies of smoking in relation to mortality has over 50 years of follow-up available [44].

What are the results of this study?

In men who reported never smoking, there was no association between smoking in the spouse and each of the three outcomes (CHD, lung cancer, COPD). First, let's look at the 'Total of current smokers' (Table 7, p.6 in the paper) which groups all the cigarette categories into 'smokers' vs. never and former smokers, from baseline to end of follow-up (the first column, labelled 'All 1959 participants, followed 1960–98'). We should focus on the 'Fully adjusted relative risk' and its confidence intervals, because the age-adjusted risk is not adjusted for the seven other confounding factors. In actuality, these figures are hazard ratios, used to estimate the relative risk of death over follow-up after censoring has been taken into account, but some authors prefer to simply call them relative risks. The relevant figures are shown in Table 9.1.

All three of the hazard ratios are consistent with no association (HR = 1) because the confidence intervals include 1. The hazard ratio for COPD suggests an increase in risk (1.28) but the hazard ratio of 0.57 for lung cancer suggests

Table 9.1 Fully adjusted relative risks (Table 7 in the paper)

	CHD	Lung cancer	COPD
Total of current smokers	HR = 0.92, 95% CI 0.80, 1.05	HR = 0.57, 95% CI 0.26, 1.26	HR = 1.28 = 0.72, 2.27

Table 9.2 Analysis of CHD deaths

CHD deaths	Number of deaths (number of participants)	Fully adjusted HR (95% CI)	Notes
1–9	81/392	0.98 (0.78, 1.24)	No association
10–19	99/513	0.82 (0.66, 1.02)	No association
20	81/458	0.89 (0.70, 1.13)	No association
21–39	27/129	1.13 (0.76, 1.68)	Threshold effect?
>=40	13/45	1.24 (0.70, 2.19)	Evidence for dose-response association

a decrease in risk; a protective effect of current smoking in the spouse. Aside from the wide confidence intervals which mean this should not be considered reliable, it could be picking up a healthy survivor effect [4]. Those most susceptible to the exposure may already have died in 1959 when recruited into the study, leaving healthier participants in the cohort. Healthy survivor effects are more common in older cohorts.

One finding that is potentially important is that above 20 cigarettes per day, CHD risk is increased and there is some evidence of a dose-response association here. This is not statistically significant, but there are relatively few people in these categories, which could lower statistical power:

These results are consistent with a 13 per cent increase in risk of CHD death when the spouse smoked 21–39 cigarettes per day, rising to 24 per cent increase in risk for >=40 cigarettes per day. Wide confidence intervals could reflect low power. A threshold effect may exist, whereby only heavy smoking in a spouse is associated with increased risk. This is consistent with what we might expect, because if there is an association, it must be weaker than for primary smoking, and is likely to be picked up at the higher number of cigarettes smoked by the spouse. The absolute risk reduction is not shown.

The authors conclude 'The relative risks were consistent with 1.0 for virtually every level of exposure to environmental tobacco smoke, current or former' (p.6) but acknowledge that 'they do not rule out a small effect' (p.9).

How precise are the results? How precise is the estimate of the risk?

As mentioned above, the results are not very precise because the confidence intervals are wide. This could reflect misclassification of the exposure (including measurement error in how spouse smoking was recorded), and low power (particularly for the dose-response results for CHD deaths). There may be residual confounding, including by widowhood. If the association between environmental exposure is small (e.g. HR = 1.05), then very large sample sizes may be required to estimate this effect precisely.

Do you believe the results?

The results show a potentially important association between heavy smoking in spouses and CHD deaths, and between smoking and COPD deaths, not statistically significant. This is consistent with expectations, because environmental exposure to smoking will inevitably have a smaller risk than that for primary smoking. Heavy smoking in a spouse is biologically plausible as a risk factor for non-smokers experiencing adverse health outcomes, including mortality. Given the relatively small number of heavy smoking spouses, and few deaths available, it is premature to draw conclusions.

Can the results be applied to the local population?

The authors suggest that public health advocates have exaggerated the claims about passive smoking. Although their study was based on a large sample of people with a long follow-up time, there were relatively few deaths among participants who had heavy smoking spouses. The effect of passive smoking could be small, only detectable at >20 cigarettes/day for example. This study was not powered to detect such an association. Even a small effect could be considered important when applied across the whole population. It would be premature to conclude that passive smoking has no association with CHD, lung cancer or COPD mortality. We also have to remember that mortality is only one endpoint. Passive smoking could be related to morbidity, self-rated health, mental health and other outcomes. Public health advice should continue to emphasise the importance of smoking cessation, or cutting down for people who feel unable to quit – for all adults.

Do the results of this study fit with the other available evidence?

The results suggest no association between environmental exposure (as measured by spouse smoking) and CHD, lung cancer and COPD mortality. This is not consistent with other evidence showing that there is an association between passive smoking and lung cancer, for example [68]. These results are consistent with a small effect at heavier levels of smoking and could reflect low statistical power arising from the small number of deaths in these categories.

Joint effect of cigarette smoking and alcohol consumption on mortality [69]

Smoking and heavy alcohol consumption may produce multiple risk of mortality, meaning that each is a risk factor. Sometimes however, the combined effect of two different exposures (risk factors) is also greater than the effect of each exposure separately. When this happens, it is called an interaction, because the two exposures do something differently when combined. For example, the combined effect may increase risk over and above any risk conferred by the exposures on their own. Interaction is also called 'effect modification', and was discussed in more detail in Chapter 6 and in several journal articles [70-73].

Here, we are going to critically appraise a paper where researchers claim to have found an interaction between cigarette smoking and alcohol consumption on mortality risk. This has important implications in public health and other disciplines, because interventions for individual behaviours may offer a double divided. When two exposures interact, removing one of them does not only remove the risk associated with that exposure, it removes any excess risk from its interaction with the other exposure [74]. For example, suppose that smoking and heavy alcohol consumption both increase risk of mortality, but their combined effect is even stronger. Smoking cessation would reduce the risk of mortality, because it increases risk on its own, but it would reduce it even further because the combined effect would no longer exist. For this and other reasons, interactions between risk factors are important to know about [75, 76]. Knowledge about interactions can improve the evidence base, and offer patients even more reasons to change their health behaviours. In the example here, heavy committed smokers who feel unable to quit smoking, might be encouraged to reduce their alcohol consumption instead. This might reduce some of the risk from alcohol and from the interaction. Interactions are notoriously difficult to replicate however, so let's first focus on whether the study actually shows evidence that these two behaviours interact.

Download this paper from http://www.ncbi.nlm.nih.gov/pmc/articles/PMC2997335/

Did the study address a clearly focused issue?

The paper seems to be clearly focused, in terms of the population, risk factor(s), the outcome and whether they tried to detect a harmful or beneficial effect:

- the population studied is husbands of women enrolled in the Shanghai Women's Health Study (SWHS);

- the risk factors studied are cigarette and alcohol consumption (and also their combined or 'joint' effect);

- the outcome is mortality, both all-cause and cause-specific (CVD and cancer mortality);

- the researchers note that smoking is expected to have a harmful effect, alcohol is expected to have a non-linear effect (moderate consumption may be beneficial, heavy consumption may be harmful) and their combined effect is not clear at this stage.

It is acceptable for a research hypothesis to be left open in this way. Because the literature about how smoking and alcohol might interact is relatively small, there may not be sufficient background in order to make a prediction about the direction of the effect.

Did the authors use an appropriate method to answer their question?

A cohort study is a good way of answering the question under the circumstances. As with the previous paper on passive smoking we appraised, it would not be ethical or feasible to expose people to cigarette smoke and alcohol, to see if it increased their mortality risk. Following a large group of people, some of whom smoke and drink alcohol, to see what happens to them, is appropriate.

Was the cohort recruited in an acceptable way?

This cohort was recruited from another cohort, the Shanghai Women's Health Study (SWHS). It is not clear why the husbands of women in SWHS were used, rather than the women in the SWHS cohort themselves. From the description under 'Methods' (p.314) it seems that cigarette and alcohol information was contained within a questionnaire for the husbands, and by implication, not for the women themselves. It is also possible that the original focus of the SWHS cohort was diet, and this is why smoking and alcohol were not originally included in the women's questionnaire. The cohort covers seven geographical regions, and is therefore likely to generalise beyond one region. The cohort being used for analysis comprises only married men. Since the biologic effect of smoking and/or alcohol is unlikely to be different in unmarried men, this is acceptable, although we should consider marital status as a potential confounder. The results will not be confounded by sex differences, because women are not included, but the interaction may behave differently in women if there are sex differences in the biologic effect of either behaviour on mortality.

Was the exposure accurately measured to minimise bias?

Both behaviours were measured by self-report. This is commonplace for large epidemiological studies, and we know that self-reports are reasonably accurate. Alcohol consumption may be susceptible to recall bias [77], and this is particularly important when looking at dose-response effects.

Was the outcome measured appropriately to minimise bias?

The survival status was available for 96.7 per cent (p. 314) of the men, which was obtained by self-report (presumably by their wives). A population-based death registry system was then used to verify the cause of death. The cause however, could be determined by medical professionals, community health workers, or legal medical experts. The accuracy of causes of death may differ according to who made the judgement. This should not influence results however, because it is unrelated to the exposures.

Have the authors identified all important confounding factors?

The authors identify several confounding factors, which we can see at the bottom of Table 2 in the paper (p. 316): age, education, body mass index, and several chronic diseases. These may be causally related to smoking, alcohol and mortality. Other confounding factors might include occupational social class and income, because educational attainment may not capture all aspects of SES. Sex and marital status are not relevant here, because the sample comprises only married men. By definition, sex and marital status cannot be confounding factors here (see Chapter 6).

Have they taken account of the confounding factors in the design and/or analysis?

Yes, their model makes adjustment for these factors.

Was the follow-up of subjects complete enough?

The authors acknowledge that they did not perform a record linkage (p. 317) for all cohort subjects. Instead, they relied only on those who were reported to have died. This means that some men may have died, but were treated as alive in the analysis. This would bias results towards 'no association' (HR = 1) leading the researchers to under-estimate any association.

Was the follow-up of subjects long enough?

Participants were followed for a mean of 4.6 years (1996 to 2000), which is not very long. The effects of smoking, alcohol use and their combined effect may accumulate over many years, perhaps even decades [44]. However, if they do find effects within such a short follow-up time, this strengthens confidence in the results because it means the effect is detectable quite quickly.

What are the results of this study?

The results are quite complicated, so we will first look at the results concerning smoking, then the results for alcohol, then the combined effect.

The results are shown in Table 2 (cigarette smoking and alcohol consumption), with some additional results on type of alcohol beverage (Table 3) and then another table, Table 4, looking at the joint effect. We will focus on Table 2 and Table 4 here. The relevant results from Table 2 in the paper are shown here in Table 9.3. For each health behaviour, we are shown the hazard ratio (HR) and 95 per cent confidence intervals for all-cause, CVD and cancer mortality separately.

Table 9.3 Cause of death (from Table 2 of the paper)

	All-cause	CVD	Cancer
Smoking status of spouse	*HR (95% CI)*	*HR (95% CI)*	*HR (95% CI)*
Non-smokers (reference group)	1	1	1
Former smokers	1.6 (1.4, 1.8)	1.8 (1.5, 2.2)	1.3 (1.1, 1.7)
Current smokers	1.4 (1.3, 1.6)	1.7 (1.5, 2.1)	1.3 (1.1, 1.5)
Non-drinkers (reference group)	1	1	1
Former drinkers	1.3 (1.1, 1.5)	1.1 (0.8, 1.4)	1.4 (1.1, 1.8)
Current drinkers	0.9 (0.8, 1.0)	1.0 (0.9, 1.2)	0.8 (0.6, 0.9)

Non-smokers are the reference group, against which ex-smokers (former smokers) and current smokers are compared. Non-drinkers are the reference group, against which ex-smokers and current drinkers are compared.

The first thing to notice is that both current smokers (HR = 1.4) and ex-smokers (HR = 1.6) have an increased risk of death from all-causes, CVD and cancer. The effect is strongest for CVD mortality (HR = 1.7 and 1.8), weakest for cancer mortality (HR = 1.3 for both groups), and somewhere in between for all-causes (HR = 1.4 and 1.6). This is in line with expectations, given that we know smoking is a strong risk factor for CVD, and also a risk factor for several different kinds of cancer (e.g. lung cancer).

The picture for alcohol drinking is more complex. Former drinkers have an increased risk of death from all-causes (HR = 1.3) and cancer (HR = 1.4). There is a non-significant trend suggesting that current drinkers have a reduced risk of death from all-causes (HR = 0.9, but the upper confidence interval touches 1). Current drinkers have a reduced risk of cancer mortality (HR = 0.8). All other results are non-significant.

Dose-response evidence provides more convincing data that an association is causal. Let's now look at the association from lower to higher levels of consumption, also shown in Table 2 but extracted in Table 9.4.

For smoking, there is a clear dose-response association from less (1 to 9) to more (>=10) cigarettes smoked, for all-cause and CVD mortality. For cancer mortality, no association is seen in the >=40 cigarettes/day group, which is surprising. Note however, that there were fewer people in this group, and also that very heavy smokers may have already died, introducing a healthy survivor effect which could bias the results.

For alcohol, the pattern is less clear. There seem to be protective effects of alcohol at the low to moderate levels of consumption, but then harmful effects at the higher levels. This pattern is a non-linear pattern, often seen by other researchers, who describe a 'U shaped' or 'J shaped' association between alcohol and mortality risk [78]. The risk is lowest for moderate drinkers, higher for non-drinkers and heavy drinkers, for example. Some commentators have argued that the higher risk in non-drinkers might be confounded by health status of non-drinkers. People may abstain from drinking alcohol for health reasons for example.

Table 9.4 Cause of death: levels of consumption (from Table 2 of the paper)

	All-cause	CVD	Cancer
	HR (95% CI)	HR (95% CI)	HR (95% CI)
Never smoked (reference group)	1	1	1
1–9 (cigarettes per day)	1.2 (1.1, 1.4)	1.5 (1.1, 1.8)	1.0 (0.8, 1.4)
10–19	1.3 (1.2, 1.5)	1.4 (1.2, 1.8)	1.3 (1.0, 1.6)
20–39	1.7 (1.5, 1.9)	2.1 (1.8, 2.5)	1.5 (1.2, 1.8)
≥ 40	1.9 (1.6, 2.4)	2.8 (2.0, 3.8)	1.0 (0.6, 1.6)
Never drinkers (reference group)	1	1	1
1–7 (standard drinks – approx 12g ethanol)	0.7 (0.6, 0.9)	0.8 (0.6, 1.0)	0.7 (0.5, 1.0)
8–14	0.9 (0.7, 1.0)	1.0 (0.8, 1.3)	0.7 (0.5, 0.9)
15–21	1.0 (0.7, 1.4)	1.2 (0.8, 1.9)	1.0 (0.6, 1.8)
22–28	1.0 (0.8, 1.2)	1.1 (0.8, 1.6)	0.9 (0.6, 1.4)
29–42	1.1 (0.8, 1.6)	1.2 (0.7, 2.1)	0.7 (0.3, 1.8)
> 42	1.6 (1.3, 2.1)	1.7 (1.1, 2.5)	1.5 (0.9, 2.6)

The authors present a p-value for the interaction which was not statistically significant ($p = 0.87$). This suggests that the combined effect of each behaviour is not significantly greater than their separate effects, and that there is no strong evidence supporting effect modification. To illustrate how the combined effect has been shown in Table 4 in the paper, Table 9.5 offers a simplified version of the results. Think about what you would expect to see if the risk of mortality was even greater when smoking was combined with heavy alcohol drinking. You would expect to see an even stronger hazard ratio for that group, shown in the box in Table 9.5. This is exactly what we see.

The results are slightly complicated by the fact that moderate alcohol drinking may be protective, so we do not see a linear increase from never, to moderate, to heavy alcohol consumer (as with the results focusing on alcohol only, in Table 2 in the paper). In both moderate smokers and heavy smokers, we see a decrease in the risk from never to moderate alcohol consumption, then an increase from moderate to heavy. This is consistent with a 'U-shaped' association. The effects are stronger among heavy smokers. In fact, what we do see is the strongest association in the combined, 'super-exposed' heavy alcohol and heavy smoker group (HR = 1.9). However, this combined effect is not significantly stronger overall, because the p-value for interaction was 0.87.

How precise are the results?

The confidence intervals are fairly narrow, reflecting the sample size and substantial number of people in each group. The results are not as precise for alcohol drinking, with many groups having confidence intervals that include or touch 1.

Table 9.5 Combined effect (extracted from Table 4 of the paper)

	Never alcohol consumer	Moderate alcohol consumer (1–21 drinks per week)	Heavy alcohol consumer (>=22 drinks per week)
	HR (95% CI)	HR (95% CI)	HR (95% CI)
Never smoker	1 (reference group)	0.8 (0.6, 1.0)	1.0 (0.6, 1.6)
Moderate smoker (<20 cigs/day)	1.3 (1.1, 1.4)	1.0 (0.9, 1.2)	1.7 (1.2, 2.2)
Heavy (>=20 cigs/day)	1.7 (1.5, 2.0)	1.4 (1.2, 1.7)	**1.9 (1.6, 2.4)**

Do you believe the results?

The results for cigarette smoking are believable, although it is strange that the effect sizes for ex-smokers are similar to those for current smokers. Since quitting smoking is associated with a reduction in risk, we would expect to see stronger effects for current smokers. The results for alcohol drinking are more complex. The fact that ex-smokers have increased risk of mortality could reflect morbidity, and the phenomenon known as 'sick quitters'. Have people stopped drinking alcohol, because they have been diagnosed with a chronic disease? This could reflect confounding by health status, although the authors did control for several chronic diseases. They also report repeating results after excluding those with chronic illness (p. 315) and say that results did not change materially. It is unclear why current drinkers have less risk of cancer mortality, although if we believe the wider literature, there may be some protective effect of moderate drinking on some types of cancer. Based on the p-value for interaction, we should not believe that the two behaviours interact, at least for these outcomes and for this length of follow-up time. Cumulative damage resulting from both behaviours may occur [76], but perhaps this needs a longer follow-up period to be detectable.

Can the results be applied to the local population?

The biologic mechanism underlying the association between smoking and mortality, and between alcohol and mortality, will be the same in men and women, and in China vs. elsewhere. The pattern of results, however, does not fit with other available evidence, (see below), so we might be reluctant to apply the results to our local population – particularly if that involved concluding that alcohol protected against cancer mortality. This may not be a wise public health message.

Do the results of this study fit with the other available evidence?

The dose-response analysis for alcohol seems to show stronger effects for moderate drinking and cancer mortality. Existing systematic reviews suggest that alcohol may be associated with oral cancer [79]. Concerning mortality, there is some evidence of a protective effect of moderate wine consumption on all-cause and cancer mortality [80], which does fit with this study. The null results for CVD mortality do not fit with other evidence, suggesting a protective effect of moderate alcohol consumption on CVD mortality [81]. In the literature however, the apparent protective effect of moderate alcohol drinking has been called into question. Does moderate drinking actually reflect SES for example, or a 'moderate personality' type? There could be residual confounding in this association. The pattern of results showing a potentially stronger combined effect of smoking and heavy alcohol consumption fits with other evidence [75, 76, 82], but is not a significant interaction here. Longer follow-up times are needed, and it would be helpful to look at systematic reviews and meta-analysis [76, 81] to see what the 'totality' of available evidence suggests.

Institutional risk factors for norovirus outbreaks in Hong Kong elderly homes: a retrospective cohort study [83]

Our final paper to critically appraise in this chapter is a retrospective cohort study.

Download this paper from http://www.biomedcentral.com/1471-2458/11/297

Did the study address a clearly focused issue?

The research question was fairly focused, asking which institutional factors in care homes for the elderly might be associated with norovirus outbreak. A range of factors were chosen, widening the focus slightly from any one risk factor. Whether these were harmful or beneficial was left open.

Did the authors use an appropriate method to answer their question?

A cohort study is a good way of determining which factors in homes for elderly persons might be associated with norovirus outbreaks. A prospective cohort study might take a long time to conduct, because this would involve noting the characteristics of each home and then monitoring whether or not outbreaks occurred over a period of time, perhaps several years. It is more practical to conduct a retrospective cohort study, as done here. The authors first looked at norovirus outbreaks across all homes, and then went back to look at the characteristics of the homes in order to identify possible risk factors for the outbreaks.

Was the cohort recruited in an acceptable way?

The units of observation were care homes, rather than the individuals living in those care homes. The study is therefore a cohort of homes, rather than a cohort of people. The research team included 748 out of 760 homes in the region, which is good coverage. We can expect this sample of homes to be representative of all homes in the region, for this reason. We might be slightly concerned that one of the homes seemed to have a duplicate ID number, which might suggest some error in the data surveillance system (p.3). Self-care hostels were excluded, because they were not comparable with standard homes, meaning that the results may not generalise to those types of institutions. They were included in sensitivity analyses however, which are reported in the results section, mitigating concerns that results would have been different had they been included.

Was the exposure accurately measured to minimise bias?

The exposures were accurately measured, although the choice of exposures is not explained. The various institutional risk factors may have been selected on the basis of previous research, or for convenience because data on them was available from the Territory-wide Infection Control Checklist Survey (described on p.2 in the paper). The researchers may have had to rely on what data had previously been collected, which is acceptable. The survey seems reasonably objective, although there is clearly room for some subjective assessment of things like 'hygiene condition of toilets and kitchens'.

Was the outcome accurately measured to minimise bias?

The measurement of the outcome (norovirus outbreak) depends on whether or not the outbreak was actually reported. As the authors acknowledge in their discussion section, outbreaks may have been under-reported by the homes. This could reduce the likelihood of finding significant risk factors in their analysis. The data came from the Public Health Information System in Hong Kong, which relies on hospital clinicians or staff from the elderly homes reporting an outbreak. If they report an outbreak, it is verified using stool samples. If they do not report it, this introduces bias because the outcome would be classified as having no outbreak (misclassification). The system has some unreliability, which is difficult to quantify. The outcome assessor was not blinded to exposure, but this arguably does not matter.

Have the authors identified all important confounding factors?

The institutional factors identified could be considered risk factors, or confounding factors. The status of each variable is unclear, perhaps because the research question is quite exploratory. None of the factors has been proposed a single 'risk factor'. This is not necessarily problematic, but it does make it difficult to think about what should be included in the statistical model. As an example, homes with more bedridden residents might have more outbreaks, but since homes with older residents have more bedridden residents, the age structure of the homes is a confounding factor. Older age may also be a risk factor in its own right. As the authors acknowledge, individual behaviours (e.g. of staff and residents) are not included because the study is only focused on institutional factors.

Have they taken account of the confounding factors in the design and/or analysis?

The authors have used a special kind of Cox Regression model to control for confounding factors. The kind of model they used takes into account the fact that outbreaks may be clustered in each home, because homes are likely to have multiple events from different people in the same home. The model they used also takes into account the fact that outbreaks are rates, producing a Poisson distribution (Figure 1 in the paper is a Poisson distribution, often seen when plotting outbreak rates) unsuitable for standard Cox regression analysis. Their model addresses both these issues. It also makes adjustments for each of the institutional factors included in the model, although as mentioned above, it is not clear which are risk factors and which are confounding factors. Another potential problem is that they explored bivariate (two variable) associations between each factor on its own and outbreaks, and then used these results to inform their decisions about what to include in the multivariate Cox model:

> Significant factors identified in the univariate analysis ($P < 0.10$) were included in the multivariate Cox regression model to further explore their relationships with the norovirus outbreak rates (p.4)

This can be problematic because variables might behave differently when considered on their own, and when considered in the full model. It is only after adjusting for all known confounders that we can arguably get a handle on what the associations are. For a discussion of this issue, see a paper by Babyak [84]. He recommends against univariate pre-testing or screening for significant associations and then 'culling' non-significant predictors prior to multivariate analysis:

> variables in isolation may behave quite differently with respect to the response variable when they are considered simultaneously with 1 or more other variables (p.417).

The authors have addressed the problem of time-varying confounding, which may occur if the covariates change their relationship with the outcome over time. For example, the age structure of a home might change over the three years of the study, or a home might become more hygienic over time if more hygienic practices have been adopted.
A similar issue is raised by the statement that,

> If two variables were believed to be proxies for similar biologic meaning, and were highly correlated with each other, the one most significant in the univariate analysis was included in the multivariate model (p.3).

The authors are correct that including highly correlated variables in the same model can introduce multicollinearity. It is often better to choose one variable, because including both can distort the estimates produced by the model (see Chapter 13 for more discussion of this). Their approach is reasonable, but the criterion of selecting the most significant variable is still a form of pre-testing or screening. It might be better to choose a single indicator that represents the intended variable beforehand.

Was the follow up of subjects complete enough?

All of the homes were monitored by the same surveillance system, meaning that follow up was complete. This study was retrospective, starting with the data and then going back to identify the characteristics of residential homes that might be associated with the outbreaks. In this situation there is no 'loss to follow-up'.

Was the follow up of subjects long enough?

Three years is sufficient time for norovirus outbreaks to occur (2004–2007) and 748 were recorded. A statistical power calculation is not provided, however, which means we cannot evaluate whether the study had a sufficient number of events to detect smaller associations than those found.

What are the results of this study?

From 2004–2007, three years of follow-up, there were $3 \times 748 = 2244$ home years and $100 \times (276/2244) = 12.3$ outbreaks per 100 home years, using whole years to calculate by hand. There were $3 \times 365.25 \times 748 = 819,621$ bed days, meaning that there were $1000 \times (276/819,621) =$ about 0.0034 episodes per 1000 bed days. The figures above use whole years rather than the number of days in each year, which will differ in leap years, explaining small differences with the figures in the paper. It is often helpful to quickly calculate figures yourself in this way, using the numbers shown (p.4 in the paper), to check that you get something nearly the same as what is reported. If we wanted to express the outbreaks in terms of a rate per person (person-years), we could take the number of infected residents/the number of residents in total = 3452/57321 = 0.06 or 6 per 100 person/years. However, the authors sensibly exclude outbreaks where one person was infected (not really an 'outbreak') which works out at 2.0 per 100 person/years.

In univariate analysis, homes with a larger capacity were 50 per cent more likely to have norovirus outbreaks, those with higher staff to resident ratios were 20 per cent more likely, those with older residents were 20 per cent more likely and those with better wheelchair accessibility were 3.5 times more likely. Home with partitions between beds were less likely to have outbreaks (RR = 0.25, which is 1/0.25=4 times less likely). The very large estimate for infection control training (RR = 3.5) and its wide CI seem strange (0.5–25.6) particularly because training is associated with *increased* risk of outbreaks, but this could reflect small cell sizes in the 2 × 2 tables, or a strong tendency for homes having undergone training to report outbreaks (a form of bias, the same problem with under-reporting mentioned above). These figures come from Table 1 in the paper and are crude RRs. As discussed above however, looking at univariate results can be misleading, because we do not know how these variables might behave in multivariate model. Many of them will be correlated with each other, requiring adjustment, and some are confounding factors for other risk factors. When you look at the main results, bear in mind that the authors have pre-tested variables using the results from Table 1, before deciding what to include in their model.

In multivariate analysis, Table 2 in the paper, each additional 30 residents was associated with a 40 per cent increase in the rate of outbreaks (RR = 1.4). Each 1/30 increment in the staff/resident ratio was associated with a 20 per cent increase, that is, having one less resident for each staff member available. Having an extra 10 per cent of residents being older than 75 increased the risk by 2.1 times, although this was not statistically significant. Wheelchair accessible homes were twice as likely to have outbreaks. Having partitions between beds cut the risk by 1.67 times. No absolute risk reduction is reported.

How precise are the results? How precise is the estimate of the risk?

Most of the confidence intervals are fairly precise, with the exception of age (percentage of residents being older than 75) which was non-significant (95% CI 0.7 to 6.1 = consistent with both a decrease in risk and an increase). The widest estimate was for wheelchair accessibility, from 1.3 to 3.2, suggesting some imprecision but still a significant association.

Do you believe the results?

The results are difficult to interpret, and we may have concerns about how variables were selected for the model, as discussed above. There are some potentially useful findings however. The authors are sensibly cautious in their interpretation and offer a balanced appraisal of their study's strengths and limitations. As they note, homes with older residents may have increased risk because they have worse infection control practices, but this could also reflect impaired immunity among older adults. Larger homes also had increased risk, perhaps reflecting more opportunity for person-to-person contact which would increase risk. Interestingly, homes with more staff per residents also have increased risk. Again, this might reflect greater person-to-person contact. More staff means more people bringing in viruses from the outside world. Having better wheelchair accessibility seemed to increase risk of outbreaks, but do we believe this? It is more likely that wheelchair accessibility is picking up another variable.

Many of the variables identified in this study as possible 'risk factors' may actually be proxies for something else – such as person-to-person contact or other vectors of transmission. Some may be confounding factors rather than exposure variables. Some may be mediators, which are mechanisms in the causal chain between an exposure and an outbreak (mediators were introduced in Chapter 6). Wheelchair accessibility could be a proxy for greater opportunity for movement by residents. If they move around more, there is more opportunity for person-to-person contact, with staff and other residents. There is also the possibility raised by the authors, that the surface of wheelchairs can carry norovirus. Wheelchair accessibility however, could also reflect other things including: investment in the home by its owners, socio-economic status of the residents (particularly income – more expensive homes might have better facilities, but also have better opportunities for social interaction, visitors etc.), age structure of the residents, health status of the residents and other factors as yet unknown. Are these homes more accessible but also better quality in other ways, ways that actually encourage more person contact? The finding that having partitions between beds greatly reduces the risk of norovirus outbreaks is believable, important and potentially useful to know.

Can the results be applied to the local population?

Any biologic mechanisms that connect institutional factors to norovirus outbreaks will be the same worldwide, so the fact that this study was conducted in Hong Kong should not matter. Cultural differences in how staff and residents interact may differ. Overall, the results suggest that person-to-person transmission is the strongest candidate for being a risk factor. Rather than use the findings to suggest that homes should be made smaller, with fewer staff, or with less wheelchair access (this would not be sensible), the findings can be used to illustrate the importance of good hygiene practices (e.g. hand washing) and reminding staff and residents that viruses can easily be transmitted between people. We should not read too much into these institutional variables (size, staff/resident ratio, accessibility) because they are confounded by person-to-person contact – probably the true causal risk factor here. Having appraised this paper, we might be encouraged to install partitions between beds or make these available, depending on their cost. This seems to be a strong protective factor against outbreaks. It would have to be balanced against possible risks, such as increasing feelings of isolation among residents. Further research should identify individual behaviours and risk factors (e.g. hygiene practices, hand washing, wheelchair cleaning) before drawing any conclusions about behavioural risk factors, not the focus of this study. A major limitation of the study was that it relied on homes reporting outbreaks. Homes should be encouraged to report all outbreaks, no matter how small, to improve the quality of future data collection.

Cohorts do not need to represent populations: a note about internal and external validity of cohort studies

Prospective cohort studies do not need to be representative of a larger population. Even if they were representative, this situation would quickly change as the larger population changed – populations are not unchanging entities [85]. A study could represent a population (have external validity) but have poor internal validity (see Appendix 7). Similarly, a study might not represent any population but have good internal validity. Examples of cohort studies that are not representative of populations but have produced valid results are [85]:

- the British doctors study, demonstrating that smoking is associated with mortality (the fact that the cohort are doctors is not relevant);

- the Whitehall II study of British civil servants, demonstrating that lower status white-collar occupations are associated with worse heart health (there is no reason why this would not generalise to white-collar occupations outside the civil service);

- the nun study, showing that people (not only nuns) who use more emotionally expressive adjectives in their writing, tend to live longer (the mechanism is not understood, but is very unlikely to be specific to nuns).

Summary

This chapter has demonstrated how to critically appraise about a cohort study, enabling you to critically evaluate its usefulness to your research. It has discussed some of the limitations of a cohort study, such as recall bias and inaccuracy which may skew the association between exposure and disease, and the length of time that may be required before researchers get their results. It is important to remember that the interaction of risk factors may increase risk overall as the effect modifier means that combined risk is more harmful than the sum of two separate risks. The chapter has raised issues about appropriate research methods, both ethical and methodological, including cohort recruitment, exposure and outcome measurement, confounding factors and follow-up. You should now feel confident to critically appraise published cohort studies, identify the limitations of an existing cohort study, evaluate the validity and utility of the results, and design your own cohort study.

The next chapter discusses the strengths and limitations of case-control studies, and approaches for critically appraising published research which uses case-control studies.

## 10

Case-control studies

A case-control study is an observational study design which allows you to compare two existing groups or subjects – cases and controls. Case-control studies are often used to identify potential risk factors in illness by identifying and comparing groups or subjects (controls) without the illness, who otherwise have similarities to the groups or individuals (cases) with the illness. For example, a comparative study of smokers with non-smokers who are otherwise similar (in age, sex, general health) might highlight risk factors for development of lung cancer. Because of its observational nature, and the often limited number of cases available, a case-control study can be less reliable than a randomised control trial.

This chapter introduces the case-control study design. It also shows you how to appraise the results from a case-control study, using three different papers. Each of the papers is different, but once again, they share the same design. As with previous critical appraisal chapters, you should print a copy of the paper first and read the paper before appraising it. As you become more experienced, you will learn to locate the essential information in a paper without having to read the entire paper. As a beginner, it is helpful to read through a paper in its entirety first. Do keep in mind however, that what the authors say in their introduction and discussion should not distract you from your mission, which is to determine whether their results actually do provide evidence for a protective/harmful effect of some exposure. The information you need is usually in the methods and results sections.

The critical issues raised in this chapter to form your critical assessment framework are similar to those in the previous two chapters.

- Did the study address a clearly focused question?
- Did the authors use an appropriate method to answer their question?
- Were the cases recruited in an acceptable way?
- Were the controls selected in an acceptable way?
- Was the exposure accurately measured to minimise bias?
- What confounding factors have the authors accounted for?

- What are the results of this study?
- How precise are the results?
- Do you believe the results?
- Can the results be applied to the local population?
- Do the results of this study fit with other available evidence?

The case studies examined in this chapter are:

- pet birds and risk of lung cancer in Sweden: a case-control study;
- association between maternal sleep practices and risk of late stillbirth: a case-control study;
- mobile phone use and brain tumors in children and adolescents: a multicentre case-control study.

Intended learning outcomes

By the end of this chapter, you should be able to:

- identify the essential features of a case-control study;
- read and understand published journal articles which report the results of case-control studies;
- critically appraise a journal article or paper describing the results of a case-control study;
- summarise the strengths and limitations of a paper describing a case-control study.

What are the essential features of a case-control study?

Case-control studies are popular when the disease is rare, when there is insufficient time to wait for a disease to develop, or where it is impractical to conduct an RCT or cohort study. Consider these three examples:

1 A researcher was interested in whether drinking steaming hot tea, rather than warm tea, increased the risk of oesophageal cancer [27]. Oesophageal cancer is a rare disease, and so a cohort study might not produce a sufficient number of cases, reducing statistical power to detect an association.

2 A public health specialist is asked by a manufacturer for immediate advice on whether a new mattress product should be recalled, because there have been reports of cases of sudden infant death by parents whose

babies have been sleeping on them. In this scenario, there is simply not enough time to develop a new cohort study, and then wait and see if the mattress is associated with infant deaths. A case-control study could be performed relatively quickly, giving more immediate evidence that could be used in making a decision.

3 A dentist is interested in whether individuals with Prader-Willi syndrome have an increased rate of salivary flow, compared to patients without the disease. Here, the 'exposure' is a rare disease, and so it would not be practical to conduct a cohort study. The dentist would struggle to recruit a large enough cohort to find enough people with the exposure of interest.

Introducing key terms

Cases

Cases are selected on the basis that they already have the disease. This part of a case-control study is relatively straightforward, particularly if the existence of several cases motivated the development of the study in the first place. A clinician in a hospital for example, might have several dozen cases of disease on her records, and be interested in whether a risk factor might have contributed to the development of the disease.

Control

An important part of a case-control study is in the selection of controls, which is achieved by a process called 'matching'. Controls are matched to cases on important characteristics, such as age, sex and geographic location. Cases are matched with at least one control, and often several controls. It is not necessary to have the same number of cases and controls. Matching reduces systematic differences between cases and controls, often thought to reduce confounding. This is often true, but note that matching can sometimes actually introduce confounding. Matching itself does not remove confounding, it simply facilitates the adjustment we can make for confounding factors in the model, which needs to comprise cases and controls. Additionally, matching on variables such as age and sex is useful even if these variables are not thought to be confounding factors. Matching can be a convenient way to create a sample, for example. It is possible to adjust for confounding factors even if the cases and controls were not matched in relation to these factors.

Odds ratios, not risk ratios

A second important difference which you need to remember, is that case-control studies cannot be used to calculate risk ratios. This is because the cases and controls are selected on the basis of having the disease outcome or not. We cannot calculate the risk of having the disease, because we cannot calculate the prevalence of the disease in either of the groups. The solution is to calculate the odds ratio, which simply compares the odds of the disease in the cases with the odds of the disease in the controls. In fact, the odds ratio was invented for precisely this kind of situation. Odds ratios have other advantages too, because they are used in logistic regression models (Chapter 14). If you want to refresh your memory about how to calculate an odds ratio, check back to Chapter 4 where they were first introduced.

Exposure measurement

Finally, an important thing to consider when appraising the results from case-control studies, is how the exposure was measured in each group. This applies to any study design – the exposure should be measured in the same way for all participants. In case-control studies however, this often does not happen. Data is not collected from the controls in the same way. This can introduce bias. Consider for example, if pregnant women with a disease were interviewed by nurses in hospitals about their smoking habits, compared to controls who returned self-administered postal questionnaires. People may give different answers to a nurse than when responding to a postal survey, resulting in their smoking status being misclassified, introducing bias.

Pet birds and risk of lung cancer in Sweden: a case-control study [38]

The possible association between keeping pet birds in the home and developing lung cancer has been mooted several times [35, 36, 39]. Researchers have debated whether early reports of an association were actually confounding by smoking or socio-economic status [35, 36, 38, 39]. People who keep pet birds tended to be from lower socio-economic groups, particularly for certain kinds of birds such as pigeons [38]. Additionally, they are more likely to smoke. Does an association between keeping pet birds and lung cancer still exist, after these confounding factors are considered? This was the aim of the authors of our first case-control study which we will now critically appraise. When you read the paper, think about the essential features of this study design: the selection of cases, selection of controls, measuring the exposure correctly and in the same way for both groups. As with all study designs, pay particular attention to confounding factors.

Download this paper from http://www.ncbi.nlm.nih.gov/pmc/articles/ PMC2352554/

Did the study address a clearly focused question?

The study does address a clearly focused question:

- the population studied is adults attending hospitals in southwest Sweden;
- the risk factor studied is keeping pet birds;

- the study tried to detect a harmful effect, motivated by prior research suggesting that bird keeping is a risk factor.

Did the authors use an appropriate method to answer their question?

A case-control study is an appropriate way of answering the research question. Lung cancer is a rare disease, and if they had conducted a cohort study, they may not have enough cases of lung cancer to analyse. The study might have been under-powered. This study does attempt to address the research question at hand. It is therefore worth continuing.

Were the cases recruited in an acceptable way?

The cases are defined fairly precisely. Look at the section marked 'Subjects and methods' in the paper (p. 1236). The authors say that patients who had been referred to hospitals with 'suspected cases' of lung cancer were invited to participate in the study. Further down, they say that these suspected cases were interviewed, and some of them decided not to participate. Some were deemed too unwell to take part. Next, suspected cases were matched with a national cancer registry, using standard ICD code 162.1 which defines lung cancer. Only cases with a verified report from a clinician as well as pathologist were classified as cases, the rest were excluded and were not used as controls either. This is an acceptable method of determining cases and it is an objective, reliable system for selecting all cases. Therefore, cases were recruited in an acceptable way. The time period was 1989–1994 which allowed the researchers to collect the data. No power calculation is reported however, which is a limitation of this study.

Were the controls selected in an acceptable way?

Controls were people who were not diagnosed with lung cancer. In the 'Subjects and methods' section, we are told that controls were 'the next person in the respective county who was of the same sex and closest in birth date in the regional population register'. This is an example of matching. The researchers have matched the cases according to sex, age (closest birth date available) and geographic area (same county). Because no power calculation was reported, we cannot determine if a sufficient number of controls were chosen, a limitation of the study. Another possible limitation is that controls were interviewed either at hospital departments or at home, whereas cases were only interviewed at hospitals. This may produce bias because the controls were interviewed in different circumstances.

Was the exposure accurately measured to minimise bias?

The exposure was measured using questionnaires, which including questions on keeping pet birds for at least six months, and the length of contact and kind of bird. This is a reasonable way of measuring the exposure, because objective verification would not be practical, although the method has not been validated to our knowledge. It is worth noting that the questionnaire did not contain information on where these birds were kept (in the house? in the garden shed?) or on the number of birds, as acknowledge by the authors (p.1238 of the paper). This could introduce error into how the exposure was recorded. If we really want to measure exposure, these questions would have been useful because people with more birds and in closer proximity will be more exposed to them. Blinding was not feasible in this study. The proposed temporal sequence (horse and cart) is correct – the researchers propose that bird keeping comes before lung cancer, which is sensible.

What confounding factors have the authors accounted for?

This information can be found on p.1237 in the paper, in Table 1 and in the paragraph 'Statistical analysis'. The authors adjust for age, number of cigarettes smoked per day, number of years smoked, time since quitting smoking, marital status, occupational social class, and diet. They decided to classify those quitting within the last four years as current smokers. One gram of tobacco was treated as one cigarette, similar to other studies [86]. They did not adjust for other measures of SES such as educational attainment and income, or area-based socio-economic deprivation. Do people living in polluted areas tend to keep more birds? It is not clear why the authors have decided to analyse men and women separately, because they did not have a prior hypothesis that the association would be different in men and women (see Chapter 6 which discussed effect modification). The authors use logistic regression which is a suitable method for adjusting an association for confounding factors, when the outcome is categorical (disease vs. no disease; see Chapter 14).

What are the results of this study?

The main results are reported on p.1237 of the paper in the text and in Table 2. In men, there was no association between keeping pet birds and lung cancer (OR = 0.94, 95% CI 0.64, 1.39) after adjustment for the confounding factors chosen by the researchers. Comparing those ever vs. never keeping pet birds, this indicates an OR consistent with either moderate decrease or increase in risk. In women, results were similarly null (OR = 1.10, 95% CI 0.64, 1.90). There was also no evidence of a dose-response association. More years exposed to birds did not increase risk, which can be seen in Table 2. If there was a causal association, we would expect more risk among those exposed for more years. This is not what we see in the table.

How precise are the results?

The results are not precise, as indicated by the wider confidence intervals surrounding the odds ratios for men and women. As noted above, there was no power calculation. If the association was small (e.g. OR = 1.10), we cannot determine if this study had a large enough sample size to reliably detect a 1.1-fold increase in the odds. Another thing you should consider is that some cases, and some controls, refused to take part in the study. They are described on p.1236 of the paper, but no comparison is made between their characteristics and those who did take part. If those taking part differed on key characteristics (e.g. bird keeping, smoking, health status), this could have introduced bias.

Do you believe the results?

As described below, the results fit with other available evidence also reporting no association between keeping pet birds and lung cancer. There were some important limitations of the study, which may urge caution before taking the results at face value. For example, there was no power calculation, no questions on the number of birds, and no questions on the amount of contact with birds. Categorising the exposure into 'ever' vs. 'never' will lose precision and lower statistical power. There was no reason to separate men and women for analysis; pooling them may have narrowed the confidence intervals.

Can the results be applied to the local population?

This study was conducted in Sweden, and there may be cultural differences in bird keeping. For example, in this Swedish sample, few people kept pigeons. Earlier studies in the UK have found pigeon keeping to be relatively common, particularly in lower socio-economic groups [37]. The number of birds which people tend to keep in the local population may be important, and the location. Do residents in the local area who keep large number of pigeons, for example, keep them outside in a shed? Do people who keep canaries and who tend only to have one or two, keep them in the living room? More precise measures of the exposure would be needed. Overall, we wouldn't be particularly worried by anything we've seen in this paper.

Do the results of this study fit with other available evidence?

We may not be experts on lung cancer, or on the literature about keeping pet birds and associated health risks. In Chapter 7, we learned how to conduct a literature review, which would be helpful for situations like this, where one case-control study is not going to have 'the last word' on an issue. Rarely can one study allow us to make a decision. It may be useful to know however, that other studies published at the same time [87] and more recently have also reported no association, even those which considered the number of birds, the method of contact and where they were kept [87]. Overall then, the results from the study we appraised fit with the totality of evidence available. To be sure, we would want to conduct a systematic review and perhaps a meta-analysis (Chapter 7). For now, there is no need to make any recommendations that people should not keep pet birds.

Association between maternal sleep practices and risk of late stillbirth: a case-control study [88]

This study attracted media interest, including from the *Daily Mail*, the *Mirror*, the *Independent* and the *Guardian*.

Journalists reported that women should sleep on their left hand side during pregnancy. Although the *Independent* and *Guardian* emphasised that the absolute risk of stillbirth was low, the overall impression given by this coverage was that of a causal, definitive link. We will now critically appraise the original paper ourselves, to see if there is evidence supporting this causal link.

Download this paper from http://www.bmj.com/content/342/bmj.d3403

Did the study address a clearly focused question?

The study does address a clearly focused question, although the specific hypotheses were left quite broad:

- the population studied was pregnant women in the Auckland region of New Zealand, 2006 to 2009;
- the risk factor studied was 'maternal sleep practices', broadly defined;
- the study tried to detect a harmful effect of particular sleeping positions on the risk of stillbirth.

Did the authors use an appropriate method to answer their question?

A case-control study is a suitable design, because stillbirth is a relatively rare event. Clearly, an RCT would not be possible because women cannot be instructed to sleep in a particular position and then the risk of stillbirth monitored. Additionally, a cohort study may not have been practical, although is certainly a possibility.

Were the cases recruited in an acceptable way?

Cases were clearly defined, as 'birth of a baby that died in utero during the antenatal or intrapartum periods'. Clinicians and hospital birth records were used for checking purposes. The geographic region was Auckland, comprising three districts, clearly defined. Deaths from congenital abnormalities were excluded from the definition, as were multiple pregnancies. A statistical power calculation was reported (p.3 of the paper). This claims that for 80 per cent power, an odds ratio of 2 can be detected from the available sample size. Overall, we can conclude that cases were recruited in an acceptable way. There was a high participation rate of 72 per cent.

Were the controls selected in an acceptable way?

The authors describe the recruitment of controls on p.2 of the paper. Two controls were selected from the same district as cases, matched according to gestation. There was nothing particularly special or unusual about the recruitment of controls. There were some potentially important differences between the cases and controls (Table 1 in the paper, which we will discuss below), but these do not concern recruitment strategy. There were no differences in the participation rate of cases and controls (described on p.3 of the paper) or in terms of ethnicity, age or parity between those participating and declining.

Was the exposure accurately measured to minimise bias?

The researchers collected data using interviewer administered questionnaire, in the weeks following stillbirth (for cases) or during an equivalent gestation period (for controls). Neither cases nor controls were told what the research question was. One of the main exposures was maternal sleep position, described a little further down in the methods section. This was recorded as 'left side, right side, back, other'. These positions were recorded for different time periods: before pregnancy, in the last month, in the last week, the [last] night of the pregnancy. The term 'last night' was defined as 'the night before when the woman thought that her baby had died or, for the controls, the night before the interview'. Other questions were asked about sleep characteristics, such as daytime sleepiness, getting up to go to the toilet in the night etc. Sleep position cannot be accurately measured without special technology, so self-report was used by the authors instead. This may introduce bias. The exposure was measured in different ways for cases and controls. For cases, there was an average of 25 days between the stillbirth and the interview, which could introduce recall bias. For controls, they were asked about sleeping position on the previous night (see p.5 of the paper where the authors discuss this). This could misclassify participants and bias the odds ratio towards null.

What confounding factors have the authors accounted for?

The researchers included questions about snoring and daytime sleepiness, as a proxy for disordered breathing, which might be considered a confounding factor if it changes women's sleep position or risk of stillbirth. Age, ethnicity, parity, social deprivation level, BMI at booking and smoking are considered possible confounding factors and are mentioned in the paper. There were significant differences between cases and controls in terms of ethnicity, parity, social deprivation, BMI and smoking (as shown by the p-values). For example, stillbirths (case) were more common for women who were obese, deprived, smoking and having high parity. These differences underscore the importance of adjusting for confounding factors in the analysis. Snoring and daytime sleepiness were not associated with stillbirth in bivariate analyses, suggesting that they are probably not confounding factors. If women with poor sleep quality tended to sleep in a different position, but it was sleep quality that

Table 10.1 Sleep position on last night of pregnancy and risk of stillbirth: unadjusted OR

	Unadjusted OR (95% CI)
Left side (reference group)	1
Right side	1.88 (1.14, 3.10)
Back	3.28 (1.46, 7.34)
Other (includes front, sitting up, both sides, unsure and don't remember)	2.00 (1.20, 3.33)

was a risk factor for stillbirth, then we might have been concerned that sleep position was confounded by sleep quality, which does not seem to be the case. In bivariate analysis of sleep position, sleeping in any position other than the left side on the last night of pregnancy was associated with an increased risk of stillbirth (fourth set of results in table 2 in the paper). The odds ratio for left side is 1 because this is the reference category (equivalent to 'unexposed'). We will learn more about reference categories (when discussing dummy variables in Chapter 13):

These odds ratios are unadjusted (the authors' term is 'univariable') meaning that confounding factors have not been adjusted for yet. This is sometimes called a crude or unadjusted association, or sometimes a basic model. The authors adjust for confounding factors in the results shown in Table 5.

There may be unknown confounding factors which are not considered, which influence both sleeping characteristics and stillbirth (e.g. underlying disease, psychiatric morbidity).

What are the results of this study?

The prevalence of stillbirth was 3.09 per 1000 births (p.3 of the paper). After adjustment for age, ethnicity, overweight or obesity, parity, social deprivation, smoking, regular sleep in daytime during the last month of pregnancy, hours of night time sleep in last month of pregnancy, and number of times getting up to go to the toilet during the last month of pregnancy, there was an association between sleeping on the back, and 'other' in the last night of pregnancy, and stillbirth. Sleeping on the right side was not significantly associated with stillbirth, because the confidence intervals include 1. The effect size is quite

Table 10.2 Sleep position on last night of pregnancy and risk of stillbirth: adjusted OR

Last night of pregnancy	*Adjusted OR (95% CI)*
Left side (reference group)	1
Right side	1.74 (0.98, 3.01)
Back	2.54 (1.04, 6.18)
Other (includes front, sitting up, both sides, unsure and don't remember)	2.32 (1.28, 4.19)

large – more than twice the risk of stillbirth of women reporting sleeping on the back or in 'other' positions.

Other results were that sleeping regularly during the daytime in the last month of pregnancy was associated with stillbirth (OR = 2.04), having more than eight hours sleep was marginally associated with stillbirth (OR = 1.71 but the p value was .05 which is technically .05 or higher), and not getting up to go to the toilet during the last night of pregnancy was also associated with increased risk (OR = 2.42). Daytime sleepiness did not increase risk but sleeping during the day did, but as the authors note in the discussion section, this is not necessarily contradictory and the two variables do not correlate. Women who were able to sleep during the day may not feel as sleepy during the day, explaining the apparent discrepancy. Given that the absolute risk of stillbirth was 3.09 per 1000 births, the authors extrapolate that sleeping on the left reduces the absolute risk to 1.96 per 1000 births, and not sleeping on the left increases the absolute risk to 3.93 per 1000 births. They do not provide a formula to explain how they worked this out, but we can use a formula called the number of patients needed to be treated for one additional patient to be harmed (NNTH) to estimate the absolute risk [89], and get a handle on how large in absolute terms this association is:

$$1/(1–OR)UER$$

where UER is the 'unexposed event rate' which is 3.09 per 1000 births (this is reported at the start of the results section on p.3). If we take 2.54 as the OR for sleeping on the back (vs. left) from their Table 4, this gives =1/((2.54–1) × (3.93/1000)) = 165 people. Therefore, 165 women sleeping on their back would be expected to result in one additional stillbirth. This may have relevance when considered at the population level.

How precise are the results?

The confidence intervals are fairly wide, ranging from just above 1 to over 6 times more likely (sleeping on the back). For 'other' positions, they range from 1.38 to 4.19 which is narrower but still quite wide. Getting more than eight hours sleep was not precisely estimated; the confidence interval is under 1 at the lower end (p = .05 exactly). A larger sample size might have allowed the researchers to detect this effect more precisely. Although a power calculation was reported, it is not clear whether this made allowances for multiple testing. The authors have conducted several different sets of results for different outcomes (sleeping position, sleeping in the day, hours of sleep, getting up to use the toilet). Some of these differences may have arisen by chance.

Do you believe the results?

In addition to concerns about multiple testing, and the rather broad research question, a major concern about this paper is the measurement of the exposure. Sleeping position, for example, is difficult to recall and report accurately. The measure used has not been validated, even on a small sample of participants.

People may change sleep positions at different times in the night, and may not remember changing positions. Although the authors report that 'non-left sided maternal sleep position' is associated with stillbirth, the adjusted results do not show this. Sleeping on the right was not associated with increased risk of stillbirth once confounding factors were considered. It was only sleeping on the back and in 'other' positions that survived adjustment. It is important to replicate the risks before making strong conclusions about sleeping positions. Without knowing too much about biological plausibility of the association, we can accept the authors' claim that 'cardiac output and fetal oxygen saturation' might be involved. However, we would wait for replications before looking for biological explanations for these results. Getting too little or too much sleep has been associated with poor health outcomes of other kinds, which the authors note in their discussion section.

An additional point which the authors acknowledge is that the timing of fetal death is unknown, making a question about the 'last night' of pregnancy obscure. The authors claim that results for the 'last month' were similar, but Table 5 does not show these results adjusted for confounding factors. A prospective cohort study might be a good next step, in which detailed attention is paid to validating the measures of sleeping position. Finally, it is important not to rule out the possibility of reverse causation. Could the outcome actually be influencing the supposed exposure? It is plausible that the death of the baby might influence the position in which women sleep, for as yet unknown reasons. This would produce an association, but a spurious one.

Can the results be applied to the local population?

Biological processes linking sleep position and other sleep characteristics in pregnant women will be the same in New Zealand as in our region. Without replicating these results however, we should wait before making recommendations about sleeping position and whether this should be modified. Sleeping in a comfortable position may have other benefits which cancel out any small increase in absolute risk of stillbirth, which remains a comparatively rare event. It may be wise to encourage women to see their GP if they experience problems with sleeping during the day, getting too much sleep, or to discuss reasons for not getting up in the night to use the toilet.

Do the results of this study fit with other available evidence?

This the first study to look at risk factors for stillbirth using a case-control design. I would wait for stronger evidence, such as prospective cohort designs, using validated measures of sleeping position. The results are potentially biologically plausible but there is not enough available evidence to make a decision at this stage.

Mobile phone use and brain tumors in children and adolescents: a multicentre case-control study [90]

Mobile phone usage has increased considerably in recent decades, particularly among children. One notable finding is that the incidence of brain tumours has not increased in the US in the past 20 years, despite an increase in the proportion of children using mobile phones since the 1990s. In fact there was an increase in brain tumours in the mid-1980s but this has been attributed to improvements in diagnostic technologies [91].

Several studies have examined the possible association between mobile phone usage and brain tumours, with few affirmative results. Given that brain tumours are relatively rare, a case-control design is a sensible way to approach this question. In the article we now appraise, keep in mind the Bradford Hill criteria for establishing a causal association (see Chapter 6), with particular reference to dose-response effects. If an association is causal, we would expect to see a stronger association for those using mobile phones more often.

Download this paper from http://jnci.oxfordjournals.org/content/103/16/1264.long

Did the study address a clearly focused question?

The study does address a clearly focused question.

- the population studied was children and adolescents (age range 4 to 17) in four European countries (Denmark, Sweden, Norway and Switzerland);
- the risk factor studied was mobile phone use;
- the study tried to detect a harmful effect.

Did the authors use an appropriate method to answer their question?

A case-control study is a suitable design. Brain tumours are relatively rare, which could make a prospective cohort study difficult. The cohort would need to be large. In some countries, mobile phone usage now approaches 100 per cent, which could result in 'empty cells' when trying to analyse the data. Imagine trying to calculate an odds ratio in a 2 × 2 table (Chapter 4) if everyone was exposed to an exposure – this would be impossible. Additionally, a cohort study could take many years to show an association, particularly if the risk accumulates over several decades. Clearly, an RCT is not practical because children cannot be assigned to use a mobile phone or not.

Were the cases recruited in an acceptable way?

Cases were clearly defined, using ICD-10 codes to classify brain tumours:

All children and adolescents who were diagnosed during the study period with intracranial central nervous system tumors and who were aged 7–19 years at the time of diagnosis were eligible to become case patients. The brain tumors had to be coded as C71, D33.0–33.2, D33.9, D43.0–43.2, D43.9, or C72.9 according to the International Classification of Diseases, tenth revision (ICD-10) to be included.

Were the controls selected in an acceptable way?

The authors selected 'two control subjects per case', matching by age and geographical region. Switzerland did not have a national population registry, so the authors used a community registry instead.

Was the exposure accurately measured to minimise bias?

Mobile phone usage was self-reported. The minimum requirement for being considered exposed to mobile phone usage was 'spoken on a phone more than 20 times during their lives' and owning a mobile phone. Owners were asked about their number of subscriptions, the start/end dates, hands-free devices, the side of head typically used, number of calls per day and duration of calls. This detail is quite useful for ascertaining dose-response information (compared to simple use/non-use of mobile phones) and for determining cumulative effects (compared to current usage only). Usage six months before the study was not considered. Regular use was defined as making at least one call per week for six months prior to the study. Hands-free devices were used to correct the information, presumably on the assumption that participants were less exposed if the phone was further away from the head. The self-reported information was supplemented by data from mobile phone operators in Sweden and Denmark.

What confounding factors have the authors accounted for?

The confounding factors considered by the authors (p.1266 of the paper) were: SES (defined as educational attainment of parents), family history of cancer, past medical radiation exposure to the head, maternal smoking during pregnancy, head injuries, wireless baby monitor usage, cordless phone usage, contact with animals, urban/rural location, siblings, birth weight, premature birth, asthma, eczema and hay fever. Unusually, the authors only included confounders in the model if the OR for mobile phone usage changed by 10 per cent or more. They cite two references to support this strategy, but it is worth noting that few researchers adopt this technique. Confounders might behave differently when considered together in a multivariate model, making it unwise to consider the impact of each confounding factor on an association separately [84]. Arguably, the markers of SES are relatively weak because they only concern parental education. The authors could have additionally considered income, occupational social class or socio-economic deprivation of the area in which they lived.

What are the results of this study?

There was no association between regular mobile phone use and brain tumours, although the OR was consistent with an increase in risk of 36 per cent (OR = 1.36). There were some non-significant trends, suggesting that greater usage increased risk: having been a phone user for a longer period of time, having longer subscriptions, making longer calls, and the cumulative number of calls. When the researchers looked for specificity of an association, they did find an association in the parts of the brain where radiation exposure would be the lowest (OR = 1.92, 95% CI 1.07, 3.44). This could have arisen by chance, given the multiple testing performed. When they looked at information from mobile phone companies, the researchers found an increased risk of tumours for those with the longest period since first subscription (OR = 2.15) which was more than 2.8 years, although they do not say if this was adjusted for age.

How precise are the results?

The 95% confidence intervals include 1 (0.92 to 2.02) showing that the association between mobile phone use and tumours is not statistically significant. This was similar for other results reported. However, the OR was consistent with an increase in risk. Perhaps the study was underpowered to detect an association (no power calculation was reported).

Do you believe the results?

Time since beginning mobile phone use was associated with an increased risk of tumours, but a dose-response association was not seen for those making longer and more frequent calls. If there was an association, we would expect to see this pattern. An important point to remember, emphasised by the authors in their discussion section, is that low-dose radiation like that from mobile phones is not known to be carcinogenic. Reverse causation may have contributed to the time since first subscription result. The authors suggest that children who had been diagnosed with a tumour may have been given a mobile phone by their parents, because they wanted to protect them and make sure that they could be contacted in an emergency. The finding that regions of the brain less exposed to radiation actually had stronger associations than those exposed to more, also suggests there is no causal association. We would expect to see stronger associations in specific regions exposed to *more* radiation. This result is probably a chance finding.

Overall, the results are believable. The study was well-designed, had high participation rates (over 70 per cent) and collected data that allowed several of the Bradford-Hills criteria to be evaluated. Although there is a biologically plausible link between radio waves and magnetic fields, mobile phone have been deemed safe by the government (see http://www.hpa.org.uk/webc/HPAwebFile/HPAweb_C/1317133827077), although there remains some concern that young children may be more at risk. Recommendations have been made for people to use them for as brief periods as possible. Mobile phones have only been used widely since the 1990s, so if there is cumulative exposure, we may require longer term studies to identify this. This study does not provide any evidence that mobile phones are associated with brain tumours. Mobile phone usage may be associated with other risks, particularly accidents while driving, which should continue to be emphasised in messages to the public.

Can the results be applied to the local population?

It is appropriate to apply these results to the local population (e.g. UK) since any biological mechanism would be the same, mobile phone usage is similar to these countries, and mobile phones are not manufactured differently in different countries.

Do the results of this study fit with other available evidence?

This study fits with other studies that also found no association. However, some studies have found increased risks among adults who use mobile phones heavily [92], and the authors also note that children may absorb more radiation [93, 94]. Given that mobile phone use is highly prevalent and is increasing, and many children use phones heavily, this should be considered a priority area for future research and we should continue to monitor evidence as it develops.

Summary

This chapter has demonstrated how to ask key critical questions about a case-control study, enabling you to critically evaluate its usefulness. It has discussed some of the limitations of a case-control study such as the problem of objective verification of measurement of risk factors.

In critically assessing existing case-control studies, the chapter has raised issues about appropriate research methods, including identification of cases, recruitment and matching of controls, identification of risk factors, exposure and outcome measurement, and confounding factors. Case-control studies cannot be used to calculate risk ratios, but can be used to calculate odds ratios, comparing the odds of the disease in the cases with the odds of the disease in the controls. The chapter has highlighted the problem of fully eradicating confounding factors and raised issues around possible variability of measuring exposure, introducing bias into the study. You should now feel confident to critically appraise published case-control studies, identify the strengths and limitations of an existing case-control study, evaluate the validity and utility of the results, and design your own study.

The next chapter develops the ethical issues raised in the discussion of recruitment and methodology in the previous chapters, by examining in more detail questions around research ethics, study design, and data management.

Research ethics and data management

This chapter introduces the concept of research ethics, and then provides practical examples of how researchers might go about obtaining ethical approval for their research. To illustrate, a real example of an application for ethical approval is presented. The Integrated Research Application System (IRAS) is frequently used to obtain ethical approval for health research, and so we will focus on questions typically asked as part of an application through IRAS. Note however, that many of the questions apply to ethical issues in general, and are asked by other kinds of ethics committees. This means that the chapter will still be useful to you, even if you have no plans to apply for ethical approval using IRAS. For example, some university departments have their own ethics committees who can approve your study. In some cases, ethical approval may not be required at all. The chapter also discusses sample size, data collection, data analysis and data management. Although they may not appear to be ethical issues, they are essential for conducting a good quality and ethical study.

Intended learning outcomes

By the end of this chapter, you should be able to:

- design a clear research question;
- understand why obtaining ethical approval for research is important;
- complete an application for ethical approval for a study;
- appreciate the importance of sample size as an ethical issue;
- plan your data collection, with particular reference to questionnaire design;
- plan your data management, including data cleansing.

Introducing key terms

Ethics is formally defined as the science of morals and principles of human duty. The British Psychological Society (BPS), for example, defines research ethics as moral principles that guide research from inception to completion [1]. Other professions that may undertake health sciences research have similar definitions.

There are four main components to research ethics:

1 *Maximising benefit while minimising harm.* This acknowledges that no research is entirely free from potential harm. Even the most seemingly benign questionnaire could have unanticipated consequences. Consider for example, if certain questions were particularly upsetting for an individual, or if the answers to certain questions were seen by others in a workplace. Many drugs have side effects, and interventions of many kinds can have unpredictable consequences. For this and other reasons, ethical research involves designing a study that maximises the value added by the new evidence, while minimising possible risks associated with the research.

2 *Respect for autonomy and dignity.* This refers to the requirement to acknowledge that participants in research are free to choose, should be treated with respect, should be informed about the nature of the study (so that they can provide informed consent, or choose not to consent, as described below), and have the right to confidentiality and fair treatment.

3 *Scientific value.* It is not ethical to produce poor quality research. Poor quality research wastes participants' time, your time, and since it is unlikely to be published, it will not make a contribution to the field. Although student projects are often designing as learning exercises rather than intended to be published, it is still not ethical to ask people to take part in research that has not been carefully designed. Study designs should be appropriate to the research question, and capable of producing data that can answer the research question.

4 *Social responsibility.* Researchers should respect individuals but also groups of people, communities and the 'common good'. Researchers should think about the impact their work might have on society and the wider public, and in some cases, the environment.

Informed consent in reserach

The Medical Research Council (MRC) guidelines on good research practice say that:

Where practicable, consent that is freely given and informed should be sought from all competent participants' [95].

Guidance on writing participant information sheets and consent forms is available from the National Research Ethics Service (NRES). Guidelines from other funding councils (e.g. the ESRC) make similar reference to informed consent, and there may be differences in how informed consent is interpreted by different disciplines. Usually, informed consent means that participants have been informed about the nature of the research. There are notable exceptions to this rule. For example, psychology research often involves some degree of deception about the true nature of the research. If participants take part in an experiment about prejudice and social stigma of people living with diabetes, for example, it may not be scientifically sound to tell participants beforehand what the research question actually was. If participants knew, they might change their behaviour and this would produce poor data. It would be essential to tell participants what would be involved in the study, but providing too much information can actually raise ethical issues if it changes people's behaviour. Poor-quality research is not ethical research – it is a waste of time and resources (for the research community and for participants). Part of the role of ethics committees is to help find a balance between research designs that are scientifically sound, and protecting participants from harm that might arise if they are not fully informed before consenting to take part.

For many research designs, informed consent is practically sought by providing a participant information sheet. The information sheet explains the research in plain English, provides contact details for the researchers involved who can answer questions about the study, and explains any risks or benefits that might be involved if the person decides to participate. Often a researcher, nurse or clinician will also be available to answer questions. For some research designs (e.g. postal or web questionnaires), this is not feasible and an information sheet should contain all the necessary information about the study.

Practical example of an IRAS application

To begin an IRAS application, go to www.myresearchproject.org.uk and click on 'Enter'.

This will take you to a starting page, headed 'Welcome to the Integrated Research Application System (IRAS)'. If you do not already have a user account, click on 'First time and new users please click here' and follow the instructions to create one.

After logging in, you will be taken to a page that displays any current or recent applications that you have been working on, or recently made. In our example, a new project needs to be created, by clicking on 'New Project'.

The next page is the IRAS Project Filter. We are asked to enter a short title for the project (as an example to illustrate the UK Women's Cohort Study 2014/15).

Is your project research?

This may seem like a strange question, given that we are applying for ethical approval for a research study! There are however, other kinds of research

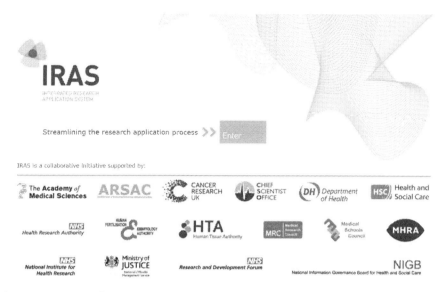

Figure 11.1 IRAS homepage

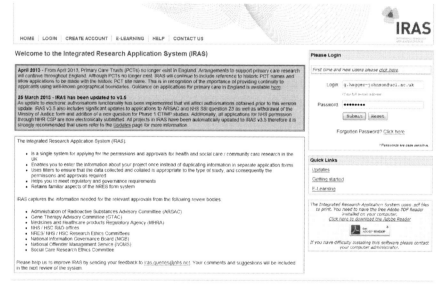

Figure 11.2 IRAS: creating an account

activity not classified as research. Audit for example, might involve analysis of health records and protocols, but may not be classified as research by an NHS ethics committee. If you are not sure whether or not your project should be classified as research, contact NRES.

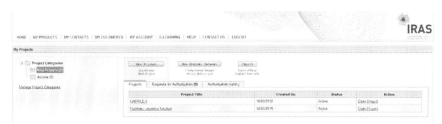

Figure 11.3 IRAS: creating a new project

Navigate | Print | Notes | Save Now | Undo

Welcome to the Integrated Research Application System

IRAS Project Filter

The integrated dataset required for your project will be created from the answers you give to the following questions. The system will generate only those questions and sections which (a) apply to your study type and (b) are required by the bodies reviewing your study. Please ensure you answer all the questions before proceeding with your applications

On-line guidance is available wherever you see a hyperlinked word or this symbol displayed. Please read this guidance carefully. For Help with your application, click here

Please enter a short title for this project (maximum 70 characters)
UK Women's Cohort Study 2014/15

1. Is your project research?

● Yes ○ No

2. Select one category from the list below:

○ Clinical trial of an investigational medicinal product
○ Clinical investigation or other study of a medical device
○ Combined trial of an investigational medicinal product and an investigational medical device
○ Other clinical trial to study a novel intervention or randomised clinical trial to compare interventions in clinical practice
○ Basic science study involving procedures with human participants
● Study administering questionnaires/interviews for quantitative analysis, or using mixed quantitative/qualitative methodology
○ Study involving qualitative methods only
○ Study limited to working with human tissue samples (or other human biological samples) and data (specific project only)
○ Study limited to working with data (specific project only)
○ Research tissue bank
○ Research database

Figure 11.4 IRAS Project Filter

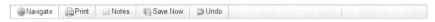

Navigate | Print | Notes | Save Now | Undo

Figure 11.5 IRAS toolbar

Select one category from the list below

This particular research study happens to involve postal questionnaires, and so 'Study administering questionnaires/interviews for quantitative analysis' should be selected.

Once you have completed this page, click on 'Navigate' to go to the navigation screen.

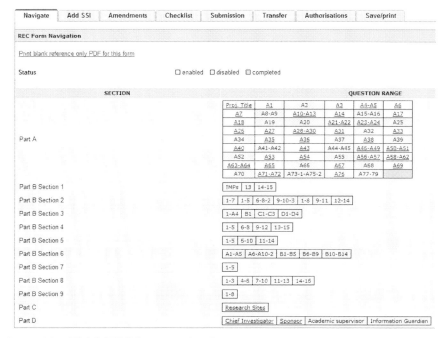

Figure 11.6 IRAS: REC form navigation

Based on your answers to the project filter, IRAS has specified which pages of the application you should fill in. These are indicated with white boxes. Questions that are not relevant to your application will be grey.

You can access the navigation page at any time by clicking on 'Click here to go directly to the Project Filter questions' under 'Project Filter' in the left-hand panel, or by clicking 'Navigate' if you are completing the application form.

Completing the application form

The application form itself is largely self-explanatory, and therefore there is no need to explain how to answer every question in detail. Some questions however, make implicit or explicit reference to ethical issues, and these will be discussed below.

Click on 'Proj. Title-A1' which will take you to page 1 of the application. This will take you to 'PART A: Core study information' where you are asked to enter administrative details such as the full title of the research, the chief investigator (usually but not necessarily yourself).

The next page asks 'Who is the contact on behalf of the sponsor for all correspondence relating to applications for this project?' To answer this question, you need to find out from your institution which person's name and contact details should go here. Check with your research and development office, manager or supervisor.

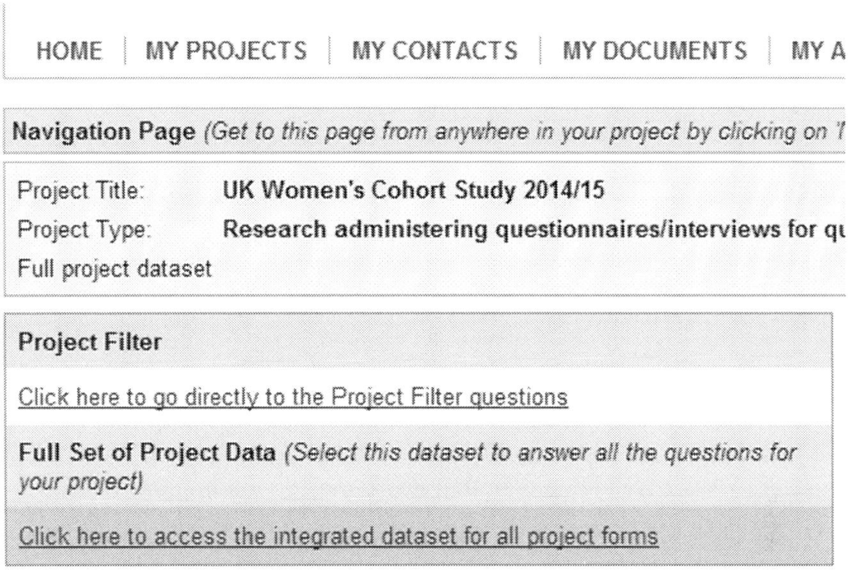

HOME | MY PROJECTS | MY CONTACTS | MY DOCUMENTS | MY A

Navigation Page *(Get to this page from anywhere in your project by clicking on 't*

Project Title: **UK Women's Cohort Study 2014/15**

Project Type: **Research administering questionnaires/interviews for qu**

Full project dataset

Project Filter

Click here to go directly to the Project Filter questions

Full Set of Project Data *(Select this dataset to answer all the questions for your project)*

Click here to access the integrated dataset for all project forms

Figure 11.7 IRAS: navigating to Project Filter questions

A5-2. Is this application linked to a previous study or another current application?

If your research study is a new study, then there is no need to answer this question in the affirmative. Many studies however, involve contacting participants from a previous study, extending a prior research project, or run in parallel with a 'parent' study. For example, our example involves adding an additional wave of data collection to an existing cohort study. This means that the application is linked to a previous study. This should be explained in the response given.

> The UK Women's Cohort was selected from responders to the World Cancer Research Fund's direct mail survey. Women aged 35–69 years, residing in England, Wales and Scotland who were willing to participate in a more detailed survey were contacted. To warrant the comparisons relating to intake of fruit and vegetables and associated nutrients and their effect on cancer and coronary heart disease, emphasis was put on recruiting similar, large numbers of vegetarians, fish eaters and meat eaters.

Three waves of data collection have taken place so far: 1995/98 (food frequency questionnaire), 1999/02 (4-day food diary, 1-day physical activity diary, familial diet/medical history), 2010/11 (follow-up questionnaire, personality assessment, online cognitive function assessment). At recruitment in 1995/98, NHS number, full name and date of birth were provided by participants in the questionnaire, submitted to the Office of National Statistics to be flagged on the NHS central register (now NHS Information Centre). Flagged participants were subsequently followed for mortality and cancer events.

A6-1. Summary of the study

Please provide a brief summary of the research (maximum 300 words) using language easily understood by lay reviewers and members of the public. This summary will be published on the website of the National Research Ethics Service following the ethical review.

This question is fairly self-explanatory, but note the importance of writing in language that the general public could understand. Applications for ethical approval will be read by a panel that contains scientists, clinicians and lay people. You must write in a way that everyone can understand what you are proposing to do.

> The UK Women's Cohort study (UKWCS) is one of the largest UK cohort studies which was set up to investigate the association between nutrition, cancer and coronary heart disease (Cade, Burley, & Greenwood, 2004). Three waves of data collection have been completed (1995/98, 1999/02, 2010/11).
>
> For the intended fourth wave of data collection (2014/15), participants will be invited to complete a follow-up questionnaire and online assessment. The questionnaire will record important aspects of successful ageing, such as self-rated health, quality of life, physical functioning, mental health and wellbeing, satisfaction with life, malnutrition, body weight, finances including 'fuel poverty'. The online test will measure reaction time, reasoning skills, memory and vocabulary. These are different kinds of mental skills, also considered an important aspect of successful ageing.
>
> As part of this wave, we also intend to recruit offspring of the UKWCS participants by asking women to provide contact details for any offspring. Offspring will receive an invitation letter and questionnaire, if their mother provided their name and address. Offspring of UKWCS will be aware that their mother provided their contact details, but will be under no obligation to take part and data will never be shared (they are linked anonymously with a secure code). This will establish a generational linkage for proposed future research on diet, ageing and health across generations.

Perhaps the most important question is

A6-2. *Summary of main issues*

Please summarise the main ethical, legal, or management issues arising from your study and say how you have addressed them.

Here, we focus on the ethical issues. Postal questionnaires rarely involve complex legal and management issues, but if you study does involve them, you also need to address that here.

There are four main ethical issues.

1 Participant burden.
Participants have been contacted three times before. As with all longitudinal research involving repeated follow-ups, participants may feel burdened. To address this, we emphasise that there is no obligation to complete the questionnaire or online assessment. Participants can withdraw from the study entirely. Participants who have already withdrawn from any previous wave will not be contacted at this wave.

2. Participants feeling obliged to take part.
When participants are already enrolled in a study, ethical issues can arise if participants feel obliged to complete any additional tasks which are proposed by the researchers at a later stage (called 'the foot in the door' phenomenon). Having enrolled at baseline, participants may not want to complete repeated follow-ups with additional tasks, but feel obliged to do so because they have already started. To address this issue, we emphasise that participation is voluntary, participants do not have to respond, and participants can request not to be contacted again.

3. Internet-based tasks.
Participants may not be familiar with internet-based tasks, possibly leading to anxiety and frustration. In 2010/11, we introduced internet-based testing for the first time to this cohort and evaluated self-rated distress and difficulty with the task, and the response rate to this part of the study as an indicator of its acceptability. Women that completed the task reported low levels of distress and difficulty, and the response rate was moderately high. We will emphasise that this task is voluntary, women can choose to complete the paper questionnaire only, and that if they feel any discomfort (e.g. due to dexterity or mobility problems) they should not complete this task. It is not described as a requirement for the study.

4. Proxy responding.
As the cohort become older, many will require help with completing the questionnaire. We observed in 2010/11 that for some participants, their partner or carer had completed the questionnaire for them ('proxy'

responding). Although in most cases women had probably asked their partner to do this, we cannot be sure that these questionnaires are 'authentic' responses. In 2014/15, an additional ethical issue will arise because the questionnaire will record several aspects of health and wellbeing which are very personal. In our view, proxy responding is not appropriate for these topics, which include psychological health, wellbeing and satisfaction with life. Women may not want their partner to know their responses to these questions, or may give unreliable responses because their partner is writing their answers down for them. To address this, we decided as a study team to ask participants to take part only if they can complete the questionnaire themselves. A message on the questionnaire will emphasise that 'you should not complete this questionnaire on behalf of someone else'. The study team will also check questionnaires on return for any indication that someone other than the participant has completed it. For example, a written comment such as 'Ella has had a stroke so I have completed this for her' would indicate a proxy response which we would exclude from the study.

5. Invitation letters to offspring of UKWCS.
Women may provide contact details for their offspring, but the offspring themselves may not wish to be contacted. Given that offspring can choose not to respond to our invitation, and will only be contacted once, in our view the inconvenience of receiving an unwanted questionnaire is relatively minor, outweighed by the potential benefit of collecting new data and establishing a generational link in the database. All new participants will be assured that no data is shared, to address any concern that personal information is communicated back to their mother.

A7. Select the appropriate methodology description for this research.

The following are ticked: cohort observation, cross-sectional study, epidemiology, questionnaire, interview or observation study. Although the original UKWCS cohort is a cohort observation, the proposed 2014/15 wave can 'stand alone' as a separate cross-sectional study, in addition to potentially being linked to previous waves of data collection. The study is also epidemiology, since it involves studying risk factors for disease in relation to health outcomes. The main method used for data collection is a questionnaire, indicated by ticking this box.

A10. What is the principal research question/objective?

Here, introduce the background to your study and state the main (primary) research question. There is space later on to describe any secondary research questions, but you may want to mention these briefly here.

People are living longer, but some people live longer and in better health than others. There is increasing interest in identifying why some women appear to age more successfully than others, having greater quantity but also greater quality of life, in the transition from midlife to old age.

Our principal research questions are:

How many women in the UK Women's Cohort Study have aged successfully in 2014/15?

What can data collected in 1995/98, 1999/02, 2010/11 tell us about why some women are ageing more successfully than others?

What new data can we collect in 2014/15 that might influence future successful ageing?

Our objective is to administer a new wave of data collection in 2014/15, involving a postal questionnaire and internet task, described below.

A11. What are the secondary research questions/objectives if applicable?

It is important not to have too many secondary research questions, because a study should be focused on one clear question. Nonetheless, there may be important questions that can be answered in addition to the main question. These should be explained in this section.

> A secondary objective is to ask women to provide contact details for any sons/daughters who might want to take part in future research. Records will be linked anonymously and stored securely, only for women and their offspring who provide informed consent for this linkage. This will build capacity for future research that will consider how dietary patterns and other behaviours influence health across generations.

A12. What is the scientific justification for the research?

This question implicitly refers to an important ethical issue, which is the balancing of risks and benefits of research. The ethics committee want to know if the research question is worth asking (the scientific justification), whether your study is of sufficient quality to be able to answer the question, and whether the anticipated benefits outweigh any risks for the participants (or for the researcher).

> Successful ageing is broadly defined as surviving into old age free from disease and disability, although many different definitions have been proposed. In a recent review of successful ageing, the three most frequently used definitions referred to physical health, cognitive function and satisfaction with life or wellbeing. Having avoided obesity can also be considered an important aspect of successful ageing, given that weight management in order to reduce the number of older adults who are overweight, obese or underweight in old age has been identified as a public health priority.

In our previous study (2010/11), we defined successful ageing among women enrolled in the UK Women's Cohort Study as reporting good physical health, being satisfied with their lives, having good mental function and having a healthy body weight. We also established that more than 60 per cent of women would provide data on mental function using a web-based task.

Although our definition of successful ageing covers four important aspects of successful ageing, there are others. In this proposed wave of the UK Women's Cohort Study (2014/15), we plan to measure a wider range of successful ageing outcomes. These include: self-reported physical health, life satisfaction, body weight, mental function, physical function, chronic disease/disability, common mental disorders, quality of life (physical, social, psychological and environment) and an overall measure of self-rated successful ageing. All of these outcomes will be measured using recognised questionnaire items, with the exception of mental function, which will be measured using an optional web-based task. In 2010/11 we only measured one aspect of mental function (reaction time). In 2014/15, we plan to measure a wider range of mental skills.

Ageing is a continuous process, and so it is important to measure additional factors in 2014/15 that might influence successful ageing in the future. We propose to measure the following in the same questionnaire: physical activity, sitting time (e.g. number of hours spent sitting watching TV), smoking, alcohol consumption, financial difficulties (e.g. fuel poverty, not having enough money for food/bills), malnutrition, leisure activities and lack of social support.

A13. Please summarise your design and methodology.

Think about whether your design is an RCT, cohort, cross-sectional or other design. It may comprise elements of both, as the example below illustrates.

The UK Women's Cohort Study is a prospective cohort study with repeated follow-ups (1995/98, 1999/02, 2010/11). The 2014/15 wave is a further follow-up, but can also standalone as a cross-sectional design. Data are linked anonymously across all follow-ups.

Participants (see inclusion/exclusion criteria) will be sent a postal questionnaire in 2014/15, with a freepost reply envelope. It will explain the purpose of the study, provide contact details for the study team, and contain clear instructions on how to answer the questions. An optional web-based reaction time task is included in the questionnaire. For participants who choose to complete it, they will be asked to go to a specified website address, complete a web-based task, and write in the results onto the postal questionnaire. To maximise the response rate, one reminder letter may be sent.

For women who provide contact details for their sons/daughters, the study team will write to each contact with an invitation to participate in the study. Existing and new data from women who provide this information will be linked anonymously only to offspring who respond and who provide informed consent to take part. The Participant Information Sheet provided to women and any nominated offspring explains the purpose of this data linkage.

A171. Please list the principal inclusion criteria

- Participated in 1995/98, 1999/02, 2010/11
- Data on physical activity and food diary
- Contact details available
- Flagged at NHS Information Service for cancer and mortality surveillance

A172. Please list the principal exclusion criteria

- Died
- Cancer registration
- Withdrawn from the study

A22. What are the potential risks and burdens for research participants and how will you minimise them?

This is another important question that refers to balancing of risks and rewards of research. Nearly all research involves inconveniencing participants in some way. The ethics committee will want to see that you have thought about this, and thought about any risks. Will you burden people with lengthy questionnaires? Will the experiment make them tired? Will they have to travel to see you? Does the drug have any side effects? Will the interview upset people?

> The questionnaire is fairly lengthy, and some participants have previously reported that they think there are lots of questions. However, discomfort associated with completing the questionnaire can be offset against the need to provide detailed information about diet, and the fact that participation is voluntary. Participants have the opportunity to see all of the questions in the survey, in a home setting.
>
> The internet-based task is likely to cause some inconvenience, and some participants may not have internet access. The inconvenience is minimised by emphasising that the internet task is optional, and the questionnaire can be returned without that information.

A24. What is the potential benefit to research participants?

Research can have benefits to participants, which might include payment for their time, being entered into a prize draw, finding out more about themselves, trying a new treatment, enjoyment, and feeling that they are making a valuable contribution to science and society. Implicitly however, this question is also asking 'What is in it for them?' Potential participants will also be asking themselves the same question! Think about what you are offering that people might like.

> Some participants report that they enjoy taking part and completing the questionnaire, because it helps them reflect on their health and well-being. Findings are communicated to participants on the study website. As with many prospective cohort studies, the benefits of participation are not always immediately obvious. However, at recruitment and follow-up we have emphasised that the scientific data generated will improve knowledge about health and disease in the longer term. We always thank women for their continued participation, time and commitment, and will continue to do so.

A30-1. Will you obtain informed consent from or on behalf of research participants?

Obtaining informed consent is an important part of most health research. Exceptions include research where obtaining consent is not necessary, but often this is better described as audit. In epidemiology and public health, population datasets such as the census or mortality records might be used for research purposes without consent. Generally, ethics committees will expect you to obtain informed consent where necessary. Obtaining a paper record of consent (e.g. with a signature) is not always necessary. For example, when people respond to postal or web questionnaires, ethics committees usually accept that people who have responded have consented to take part. You must obtain informed consent if you plan to use an intervention or experiment in your research (see Appendix 5: Consent Form).

A57. What is the primary outcome measure for the study?

This is one of the most important questions, but if you have more than one outcome, it can be difficult to answer. Usually there is a primary outcome, meaning the outcome variable you are most interested in. For trials this is usually clear, because the intervention is designed to change this outcome. For cohort, cross-sectional and several other research designs, you may be interested in several outcomes. It is commonplace for several outcomes to be analysed separately in a prospective cohort study, for example. It is good practice however, to design a study with at least one clear outcome, and use this to help you determine sample size. Ethics committees will not be impressed if you have no clear outcomes in mind, or seem unable to determine which of your variables are exposures/predictor variables and which are outcomes. In the example, meeting the criteria for successful ageing is a primary outcome.

> The proportion of women meeting the criteria for successful ageing

A58. What are the secondary outcome measures?

If you have other outcome measures, this is the place to describe them. In the example, the secondary outcomes are the specific components of successful ageing. The overall measure of success would be analysed first, and then its individual parts. Additionally, the researchers wanted to collect contact details for sons/daughters of women enrolled in the study. The proportion of women providing such details is considered a secondary outcome measure in this study.

> The proportion of women qualifying for specific components of successful ageing (i.e. each indicator separately).
> The proportion of women who provide contact details for sons/ daughters, and the response rate for these offspring.

A60. How was the sample size decided upon?

At first sight, you may not think that this question is about ethics. What does sample size have to do with ethics? In fact, deciding a sample size is a very important part of an ethical research study. This is because sample sizes determine the statistical power of a study. Miles has argued 'power is not just a statistical or methodological issue, but an ethical issue' [96]. Participants in health research are giving up their time in the hope that this will help reduce disease and disability in the future. A sample size that is too small will be under-powered, reducing the likelihood that a true effect is found. A sample size that is too large is a waste of time and resources. Why recruit too many people when you can estimate the right number of people needed to find an effect? If you do not have a statistician or someone to help you perform a power calculation, there are several good software packages available and various web resources. Additionally, there are books dedicated to statistical power analysis, some of which are listed at the end of this chapter. When thinking about sample size and statistical power, it may be important to think about clinical significance and minimally important difference (MID).

> The sample size of 3721 is based on a detectable odds ratio of 1.30, a proportion of cases in the 'exposed' group of 0.15, and a 'disease' prevalence rate of 0.48. This estimate is illustrative and based on data from the cohort at 2010/11 and a modest effect size. In reality, models will be run for more than one outcome and all available data will be used, so the analytic sample size will vary. Assuming a response rate of

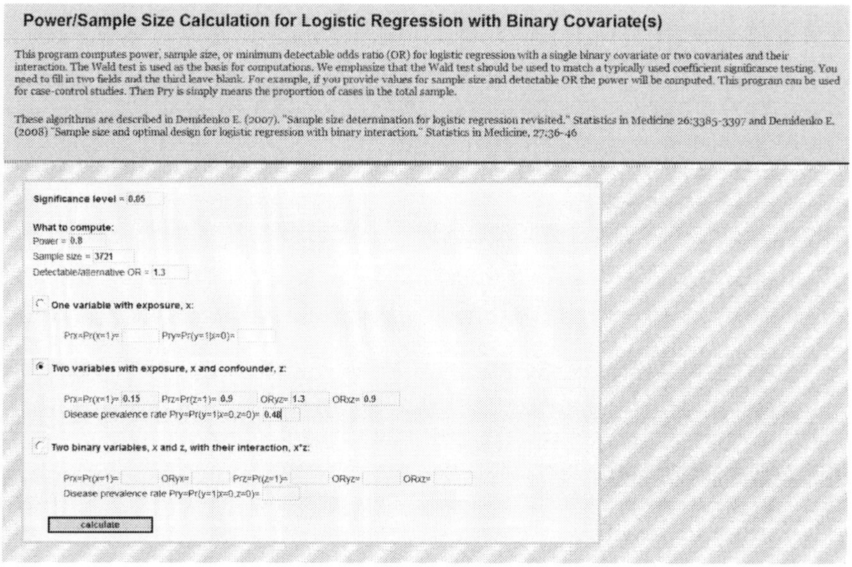

Figure 11.8 Power/sample size calculation (http://www.dartmouth.edu/~eugened/power-samplesize.php)

45 per cent, mailing 9000 questionnaires should achieve 4050 responses, although this is likely to be closer to 3700 because the cohort are older than at 2010/11.

> **A62. Please describe the methods of analysis (statistical or other appropriate methods, e.g. for qualitative research) by which the data will be evaluated to meet the study objectives.**

Ethics committees want to know how you will analyse your data. You may think that statistical analysis is a statistical rather than an ethical issue, but remember that poor-quality research is unethical research – it wastes time and resources. If you appear to have no clue how you will analyse your data, are you really ready to conduct your study? It helps to give at least some indication of the kinds of methods you will be using. For many quantitative study designs, regression models and methods related to regression (including ANOVA) will be expected. If you plan to use more unusual methods, the committee may want to see more detail. It may help to say how you will do descriptive analyses (e.g. chi-square tests, t-tests).

> Data will be analysed using logistic regression (categorical outcomes) or linear regression (continuous outcomes).

You will be expected to submit regular progress reports, notify the committee of any delays, and submit a final report. Things can get delayed, which is not problematic, but it shows evidence of good planning if you have a clear end point in mind. Research that could apparently run indefinitely is unlikely to be perceived favourably.

Planned start date: 01/01/2014
Planned end date: 31/12/2015

Informed consent in the IRAS application

The guidance notes in the IRAS application form note that ethics committees are increasingly asking, 'Can you, or whoever will seek consent, assess capacity and do you understand the ethical principles underpinning informed consent?' This raises a related but different issue to informed consent, that of capacity.

Capacity

The Mental Capacity Act (2002) requires researchers to consider whether potential participants actually have the capacity to provide informed consent for research. Some patients may not, and so special arrangements will need to be made (e.g. with carers and relatives) if you want them to take part in your research.

Other things ethics committees may ask for include:

- *Study protocol.* This is a concise summary of what will happen in the study – to whom, how many times, and in what order. It is good practice to have a study protocol before you start writing the ethics form, not least because it helps you get clear in your own mind what your study will actually involve

- *Participant information sheet.* This is an information sheet for participants, usually written in question and answer format.

- *Consent form.* Often following the information sheet, the consent form is a written and signed record that the participant has agreed to take part in the study as described in the information sheet. For anonymous surveys however, ethics committees may not consider this necessary. Returning a questionnaire can act as a proxy for providing consent – if people did not want to take part, they probably wouldn't return it. An example of a consent form is provided in Appendix 6.

- *Questionnaire or other data collection methods.*

Questionnaires

The best advice about designing a new questionnaire is arguably, not to do it! If you can possibly avoid it, it is nearly always better to use an existing, validated measure of the variables you are interested in.

If you use an existing questionnaire, scale, measure or question

- Check that the measure(s) is(are) reliable (i.e. internally consistent, and stable when administered repeatedly / test-retest reliability).

- Check for evidence that the measure has been validated (measures what it claims to measure).

If you must design a new questionnaire

- Make absolutely sure that there are no existing questionnaires, scales, measures or single questions which you can use – check, for example, the Survey Question Bank at the UK Data Service (http://ukdataservice.ac.uk).

- Creating a new measure is highly challenging, because you have to demonstrate reliability and validity yourself, before people appraising your results will accept your findings.

- Think about how you will show reliability (e.g. Cronbach's alpha for internal consistency reliability, repeated the questionnaire on a sub-sample of participants three months later, to provide test-rest reliability).

- Think about how you can demonstrate validity (e.g. showing that your measure correlates with things you would expect it to, and does not correlate with things you do not expect it to correlate with).

- You need to study guides to questionnaire design before launching into your own.

- Choose closed questions (e.g. choose from the following options: always, sometimes, never) if you want people to complete the questions quickly, and to save time at the data entry stage.

- Choose open-ended questions if you want people to express their own views in their own way, and you are not concerned about the additional time their answers will take to code and analyse. Open-ended questions may require qualitative methods in order to analyse the data.

- Think carefully about the participants' literacy and numeracy levels. Might visual scales or pictures be more appropriate than complex numerical response options?

- Check the readability of your questionnaire. For example, use MS Word to calculate a Flesch-Kincaid reading score (under the Review tab,

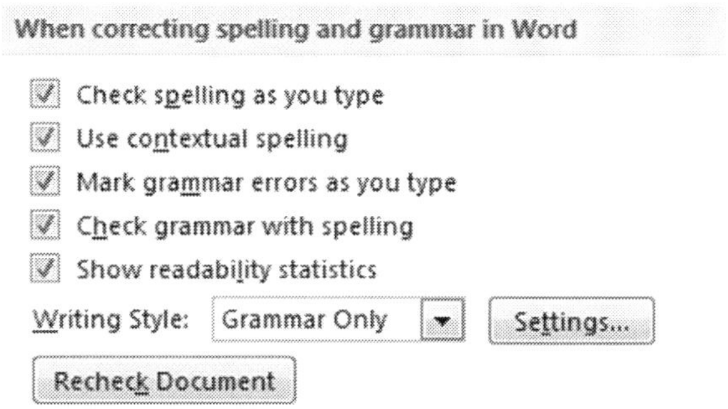

Figure 11.9 Selecting readability statistics in Word

click on Spelling & Grammar, Options, Tick the box 'Show readability statistics' under 'When correcting spelling and grammar in Word')

- Pilot your questionnaire before starting the data collection. Do people understand the questions and layout? Do they tend to miss particular questions? Should the design be improved?

Questionnaire design

Table 11.1 is reproduced from a series of three guides to questionnaire research published in the BMJ [97–99]. It is worth reading these guides if you plan to design a questionnaire yourself.

Data management

Good data management involves keeping detailed records of everything you do during the research project. If you are storing personally identifiable information, you need to comply with current data protection legislation. If you are conducting research at a public institution, or have a contract with a public body, then you should be prepared to share any information (except information that is personally identifiable or exempt for other reasons) in response to any 'Freedom of Information' request.

Data protection

You must ensure that your data collection meets the requirements of the Data Protection Act 1998. In particular, you need to check where and how to store any personally identifying or sensitive information. Check with your data protection officer to find out more.

Freedom of Information (FOI)

Any member of the public can request information about your study, including protocols, emails between you and colleagues, meeting notes and so on. Your research may be funded by a public body, and be conducted at a

Table 11.1 Guidelines for questionnaire design (adapted from [97–99])

Section	Quality criterion
Title	Is it clear and unambiguous?
	Does it indicate accurately what the study is about?
	Is it likely to mislead or distress participants?
Introductory letter or information sheet	Does it provide an outline of what the study is about and what the overall purpose of the research is?
	Does it say how long the questionnaire should take to complete?
	Does it adequately address issues of anonymity and confidentiality?
	Does it inform participants that they can ask for help or stop completing the questionnaire at any time without having to give a reason?
	Does it give clear and accurate contact details of whom to approach for further information?
	If a postal questionnaire, do participants know what they need to send back?
Overall layout	Is the font size clear and legible to an individual with 6/12 vision? (Retype rather than photocopy if necessary)
	Are graphics, illustrations and colour used judiciously to provide a clear and professional overall effect?
	Are the pages numbered clearly and stapled securely?
	Are there adequate instructions on how to complete each item, with examples where necessary?
Demographic information	Has all information necessary for developing a profile of participants been sought?
	Are any questions in this section irrelevant, misleading or superfluous?
	Are any questions offensive or otherwise inappropriate?
	Will respondents know the answers to the questions?
Measures (main body of questionnaire)	Are the measures valid and reliable?
	Are any items unnecessary or repetitive?
	Is the questionnaire of an appropriate length?
	Could the order of items bias replies or affect participation rates (in general, put sensitive questions towards the end)?
Closing comments	Is there a clear message that the end of the questionnaire has been reached?
	Have participants been thanked for their co-operation?
Accompanying materials	If the questionnaire is to be returned by post, has a stamped addressed envelope (with return address on it) been included?
	If an insert (eg leaflet), gift (eg book token) or honorarium is part of the study protocol, has this been included?

university or college. This makes you accountable for what you do, and you should be prepared to share anything that would pass the 'public interest test'. The Freedom of Information Act is designed to promote transparency and accountability, which should help improve decision-making. The Information Commissioner's office say we should be moving away from 'need to know' toward 'the right to know', toward a new culture of openness [100]. You should be prepared to be transparent and accountable when undertaking research. FOI should not be confused with data protection, which concerns personally identifiable information. Following a FOI request, personally identifiable information is often removed because it is one of the exceptions to FOI (data protection requires that personal information not be disclosed). Check with your local FOI officer for information.

Databases

You may store your research data in any number of formats (e.g. Excel, Access, R, SPSS, SAS, STATA), but do remember the following:

- Personally identifiable and sensitive data should be stored separately in a secure database.

- Even when data are anonymised or linked-anonymised (an ID number could be used to link data back to named participants in a separate database), certain combinations of variables could be used to identify people. In a sparsely populated area, for example, simply knowing the job title and age of a participant might be sufficient for someone to identify them. Think carefully about the level of detail you actually need.

- Participants should have been informed if you plan to share data, and provided consent to do this. Will you share the anonymised data? Will you pass on personal details to other researchers? Will you remove some variables to reduce the risk of identification? These are all important questions that should be answered before you start the study, and they should all be clearly explained to participants so that informed consent is truly informed.

Data cleansing

Here are some tips for checking that your data have been entered correctly:

- Check the minimum and maximum for each variable. Are there any variables out of range?

- If there is a blank cell, is this a data entry error or a true missing value? It is better to assign missing values with a specific number (e.g. 9999) to make it clear that the value is actually missing. Do not forget however, to specify that this value should be treated as missing in your software package. If you do not, it will treat 9999 as a numeric value.

- If you have time/funding, do data entry twice ('double data entry') to allow checking for any inconsistencies.

- Keep the original data or questionnaires in case you need to refer back to them.

- Check that all variables are labelled correctly, that you know what each value means, and what the units are (e.g. litres, fluid ounces).

- Create a 'data dictionary' or coding book which describes all of the variables, their labels and their possible values. This will help you and others who might use the data for future analysis.

- Check for outliers (very low or very high values) and refer back to original questionnaires or raw data, to find out if this was a data entry error or a true value.

- Enter data gradually, rather than waiting for all questionnaires to be returned, for example. It will reduce the burden on the person doing the data entry.

- Save data with a new file name ('save as...', rather than 'save') each time you work on the dataset, preferably with the date. For example, if I was entering data across three days, I might end up with three files like this:

  - 2013_07_06_data

  - 2013_07_05_data

  - 2013_07_04_data

  This means that should a mistake be made, it is easy to go back to the previous file and remember which date it was created on. You can also sort the files by date, to quickly identify the newest one.

Summary

You should not underestimate the time involved in planning your research, which includes writing a study protocol, submitting your study for ethical approval, data entry, data checking and data management. Even small-scale studies take considerable time, even before you can start analysing the data.

This chapter has demonstrated the importance of a clear primary research question in focusing your research and identifying the key objectives and outcomes of your study. The chapter has raised related methodological issues such as study protocol, sample size, data collection, data analysis and data management which will help you to design your research project, but also to consider the ethical implications. As a researcher, particularly in the health sciences, you have a moral duty towards your research subjects, which involves maximising benefit while minimising harm, respecting the autonomy and dignity of research participants, ensuring the quality and value of your research, and social responsibility towards the wider public. This latter point underlines the ethical importance of research design factors such as sample size, which affects the statistical power of a study and its practical application.

The chapter has discussed the MRC guidelines on good research practice and stressed the importance of informed participant consent, as well as ethical issues around participant burden in a longitudinal study, difficulty in responding, and proxy responding. It has offered a step-by-step practical demonstration of how to use the IRAS application system which gives you a good model for identifying key methodological and ethical issues in your study design. It has also raised issues around the advisability of designing a questionnaire for your study when there may be existing questionnaires which you could use. Data management is also an ethical issue, particularly where you are storing personal information and the chapter has raised the issue of data protection legislation which may affect your research design.

You should now feel confident about identifying the main ethical issues in your study, completing an application for ethical approval for a study, and anticipating the issues in research design, data management, data analysis, and ethical questions which ethics committees may raise.

Good study design is vital if you are to seek publication of your research, which is important for your career progression and professional development. The question of practical applications of your research leads us to the importance of distributing and publishing your work, which the next chapter now considers.

## Part IV

Conducting new research

12

Dissemination and publication

Sooner or later, you may think about preparing your results for publication in a scientific paper. This section briefly reviews the different kinds of papers published by health scientists, and then shows how you might write a manuscript and prepare to submit the manuscript to a peer-reviewed journal.

Intended learning outcomes

By the end of this chapter, you should be able to:

- identify different ways of disseminating your results;
- avoid plagiarism and possible conflicts of interest;
- understand the importance of acknowledging your sources;
- prepare your results for publication;
- identify suitable journals where you can submit a manuscript.

Types of published writing

Research articles

Research articles make up the majority of published academic writing and are used to disseminate the results of original research. In the critical appraisal chapters, we appraised several examples of original research articles that had been peer-reviewed and published in academic journals. Research articles in the health sciences are typically 2500 to 5000 words in length, although social sciences and psychology tend to be longer. More medical disciplines tend to have shorter introductions than psychology, for example, where longer introductions provide more room to discuss theoretical background and introduce psychological constructs referred to in the paper.

Review articles

As we saw in Chapter 7, review articles summarise several existing research articles, to provide an overview of the 'totality' of available evidence that has been published. Review articles are particularly useful when there have been many studies published on a topic and the reader would like to orient themselves to the area without having to read all of the existing studies. Review articles are divided into two kinds – narrative reviews and systematic reviews. Narrative reviews provide a 'story' of the research but the papers are selected by the author as they see fit. Systematic reviews specify a set of criteria showing how the research databases were searched, the search terms used, which studies would be included, which would be excluded, and how results would be synthesised. It is generally thought that systematic reviews give a less biased account of the literature than narrative reviews, because an author writing a narrative review could 'cherry pick' only those articles which they thought were most interesting. Narrative reviews can be quite subjective, and give a misleading impression of the evidence base. Systematic reviews however, do not necessarily provide a complete account because the evidence reported depends on the criteria used to select the studies. If the author used a different set of criteria, they would end up with a different review. The criteria selected also involve some degree of subjectivity and personal preference.

Meta-analysis

It is important not to confuse systematic reviews with meta-analysis. Meta-analysis usually follows systematic review, but not always. Meta-analysis involves combining the results of several studies into a single summary result or effect size, and with confidence intervals. The studies may have been selected using systematic criteria, but not necessarily. An author may choose to conduct a meta-analysis of several studies simply because they had access to the results for those studies. Another author might choose to conduct a meta-analysis on all of the published results on a topic. Systematic reviews followed by meta-analysis arguably provide better quality evidence that either narrative reviews or meta-analysis without a systematic approach to choosing studies. In recent years, meta-analysis of individual participant data (MIPD) has become popular. This involves a researcher collecting the original data and then analysing all of the studies simultaneously, to produce a summary result. Traditional meta-analysis involves synthesising the existing results, usually but not always published results, from the studies. There is much greater control in MIPD because researchers can choose which variables to control for, how results are presented, and consider effect modification. Decisions made prior to publication of the original studies can be revisited in MIPD, which is an attractive feature.

Letters

Letters to the editor are short opinion pieces, often reacting to published research articles. Letters pages are an arena for debate and discussion. If a reader disagrees with the interpretation made by an author concerning their results, or has reservations about the methods used, then a letter is a suitable method for communicating these views. Letters may suggest additional confounding factors that authors did not consider, alternative ways to analyse the data, or different conclusions that could be made. Letters are typically very short, and are submitted for publication very soon after the research article they refer to is published.

Book reviews

Given that there are so many academic books being published each year, it is often helpful to read book reviews. Book reviews are written by readers of the journal they appear in, which is helpful because the review is written by someone working in a similar discipline to yourself. Book reviews typically give an overview of what the author(s) included, the structure of the book, strengths, weaknesses and a recommendation about suitable audiences. For example, the review might suggest that students should be told to read the book as part of a course.

Cohort profiles

The *International Journal of Epidemiology* has published many cohort profiles in recent years and this type of paper is proving increasingly popular. Cohort profiles provide background information about a cohort, such as when the cohort was recruited, the types of people in the cohort, what has been measured and when the cohort were followed up. This means that authors presenting results from a cohort do not need to provide a detailed description of the cohort in every paper – they can simply cite the cohort profile. Cohort profiles are an excellent way of familiarising yourself with new and on-going cohort studies.

Case reports

Case reports are common in the medical sciences, and consist of a single patient or 'case' being described to the readers. Typically this is an unusual case, perhaps of a rare condition or presentation, but not necessarily. A rare case does not in itself mean that a case report should be published – a common disease with a particularly unusual presentation or set of symptoms might also be worth publishing as a case report. A case report includes a description of the patient, the sequence of events, and what the clinician did to manage the case. Sometimes photographs are included but care should be taken to ensure confidentiality, and ideally informed consent from the patient should have been given. The purpose of case reports is typically to educate readers, and so publication in a relevant speciality journal is necessary.

The structure of original research articles

Original research articles typically follow a classic structure called 'IMRaD' – Introduction, Methods, Results and Discussion. An abstract of the paper will be presented at the start of the article and in research databases.

Abstract

Abstracts are 200–300-word summaries of the article and can be described as a miniature version of the article itself. Structured abstracts have the same headings that appear in the paper (introduction, methods, results and discussion) for this reason. Often, the abstract is the only part of the paper that will be read. Many readers will search databases for relevant articles and only read the abstract. Therefore, it is essential that abstracts are clear, concise, and include the most important information.

Introduction

The purpose of the introduction section is to briefly introduce the topic, summarise the previous research in the area, clarify an important gap in the evidence base, and propose a research question which fills the gap. When planning an introduction section, imagine a funnel shape – start fairly broad, and then end the introduction with a narrow, specific focus on the research question which your paper will address. In the health sciences, introduction sections are quite short. You can cite previous research and if available, review articles, which allow readers who want to learn more about the topic to find relevant references. Good introductions identify what the paper will add to the evidence base. They answer the question 'why does this paper need to exist?' Although replicating research findings is important, few editors of journals will want to publish an article that simply repeats what has been found already. An original research article will 'move the field forward'. Although it can raise new questions, it should answer at least one important question. When writing an introduction section, resist the temptation to provide a detailed narrative review of the field. Although you should have read the relevant papers before starting your own study, it is not necessary to cite all of these papers simply to show the reader that you have read them. Cite references selectively, focusing on key papers, more recent findings, and review articles. Introductions typically end with a clear statement of the gap in the existing evidence base and the research question which will be answered. Here are some examples:

- The concept of "lung age" (the age of the average person who has an FEV_1 equal to the individual) was developed in 1985 as a way of making spirometry data easier to understand and also as a potential psychological tool to show smokers the apparent premature ageing of their lungs. We tested the hypothesis that telling smokers their lung age would lead to successful smoking cessation, especially in those with most damage [57].

- As keeping birds is fairly common in Sweden, a relative risk of the magnitude reported in any of these earlier studies could have a substantial impact on the nation's public health. We therefore included questions concerning bird ownership in our population based case-control study of lung cancer conducted in the city of Gothenburg and counties of Bohus and Alvsborg in southwest Sweden [38].

- Although the individual effects of smoking and alcohol consumption on mortality have been well established, the joint effect of these two lifestyle factors on mortality remains unclear (Ebbert et al., 2005; Martelin et al., 2004; Yuan et al., 1997). We took advantage of the data collected in the Shanghai Women's Health Study (SWHS) about the lifestyles and health conditions of husbands of the cohort's married women and prospectively examined the relationship between cigarette smoking, alcohol consumption and mortality of the husbands. In this husband cohort, many participants were both cigarette smokers and alcohol drinkers, providing us with a good opportunity to evaluate the effects of the interaction between cigarette smoking and alcohol intake on mortality [69].

Methods

The methods section describes the methods used by the researchers. Ideally it should provide enough information to allow readers to repeat the procedure, if they wanted to replicate the study. The methods section should cover who, where, when, why (inclusion/exclusion criteria) and how. Additionally, it is necessary to provide information about who provided ethical approval for the study. For example, 'The study was approved by the University College London and University College London Hospitals Ethics Committee' [52]. Depending on the journal, methods sections are sometimes divided into further sections: design, participants, measures, procedure, statistical analysis.

Design

Describe the type of research design (e.g. RCT, cohort, case-control, cross-sectional). For cohort studies, it is worth describing the cohort briefly, and citing a cohort profile (if available) or an earlier paper which contains more detail on the cohort, recruitment, baseline measures and so on. For example:

> The Whitehall II study is based on employees of the British Civil Service [101]. At study inception (phase 1, 1985–1988), 10 308 participants (67% men) underwent a clinical examination and completed a self-administered questionnaire. Subsequent phases of data collection have alternated between postal questionnaire alone (phases 2 [1988–1990], 4 [1995–1996], 6 [2001], and 8 [2006]) and postal questionnaire accompanied by a clinical examination (phases 3 [1991–1994], 5 [1997–1999], 7 [2002–2004], and 9 [2007–2009]). [102]

Participants

The participants section describes who was included, and why. Any inclusion/exclusion criteria should be specified. For example:

> From September 1995 to November 1997, we invited homosexual men attending a sexual health clinic in London to enter the trial if they presented with an acute sexually transmitted infection, reported having had unprotected anal intercourse with a partner of different HIV status in the past year, or expressed concern about their sexual practices. Men were only excluded if they were deemed by clinic staff to be unsuited for a group education and counselling intervention. Participants were randomly allocated using sealed opaque envelopes. [52]

Measures

Information about the exposure, outcome and covariates should be provided here. For example, in this paper, the exposure was sitting time and the outcome was mortality:

> Exposure assessment. The amount of time participants spent sitting during work, school, and housework was obtained from the lifestyle questionnaire. Participants were asked to indicate the amount of time they spent sitting during the course of most days of the week as either 1) almost none of the time, 2) approximately one fourth of the time, 3) approximately half of the time, 4) approximately three fourths of the time, or 5) almost all of the time [103].
> Ascertainment of mortality. The CFS database was linked to the Canadian Mortality Database (CMDB) at Statistics Canada. The CMDB contains all recorded deaths in Canada since 1950 and is regularly updated using death registrations supplied by every province and territory. [103]

Statistical analysis

This section describes the statistical techniques used to analyse the data. Normally this includes basic descriptive statistics used to describe the study variables, and will include *t*-tests for continuous variables and chi-square tests for categorical variables. For example, tables may be presented in the results section which compares study variables across exposed or unexposed participants. The descriptive statistics should compare whether the exposed and unexposed participants differ significantly. For RCTs, baseline differences should be evaluated and any significant differences evaluated. Next, describe the techniques used for the main analysis. These might include linear regression, logistic regression, Cox regression or ANOVA, for example. Finally, describe any sensitivity analyses conducted. Sensitivity analyses are important because they evaluate whether certain aspects of the data might have influenced results. For example, a small number of participants with extreme values or deaths which occurred very soon after baseline, might have generated spurious results. If you repeated analyses after excluding these people, explain this here. In this section, do not report the results of any analysis, simply describe the methods used.

For example:

> We used a proportional hazards regression model to examine the relation between cigarette smoking, alcohol consumption at recruitment and subsequent risk of death. [69]

Results

Results are the most important part of a research article. Having said that, we saw in the critical appraisal chapters that the methods section is arguably what should be appraised first. If the methods are not suitable for answering the research question, then the results are not worth reading. Results sections are usually divided into two main sections, descriptive statistics and then the main analysis. The main analysis where the 'inferential statistics' are presented, typically involving regression models, ANOVAs or other multivariate models.

Descriptive statistics

Descriptive statistics are usually presented in the first table of a research article. Typically, each study variable is listed in the rows of the table. Researchers often use the columns to divide the analytic sample according to exposure status (for cohort studies) or treatment status (for RCTs). Cross-sectional studies might be divided into men and women, different socio-economic groups, or some other relevant grouping. Taking cohort studies as an example, the purpose of presenting statistics separately according to exposure status is to show the reader what the 'crude' bivariate differences look like, before any adjustments have been made. Are those in the highest blood pressure tertile also more likely to smoke? Is the mean age of heavy alcohol drinkers higher than moderate drinkers? Are there more men diagnosed with clinical depression than women? These are the sorts of questions which the reader is likely to be asking, as they scan your table of descriptive statistics.

- Tip: when preparing a research article, start with Table 1. Clear and neatly presented tables influence the perceived quality of a paper, help reviewers understand the data quickly, and allow reviewers to check aspects of your work. Additionally, they may help you write the paper. It can be useful to have tables beside you as you write, so that you can refer to them easily. After publication, tables will help readers understand what you have done – which is ultimately the most important feature of a paper.

Given what we have learned about confounding, you should realise that simplistic bivariate relationships presented in such tables are not necessarily informative because they can be influenced by confounding factors. They are very important however, because they can show which variables are associated with exposure status, and therefore, which might be important to control for in the main analysis. Similarly, some authors present tables grouped according to the outcome status, which also provides information about possible 'confounding structures' in the data. In the case of RCTs, comparison of study variables according to treatment status tells the reader if randomisation has been successful. If randomisation was unsuccessful, we will see significant differences between the groups at the start of the study.

Table 12.1 is an example of a table of descriptive statistics, taken from a prospective cohort study of older men [104]. The exposure is depression status (no depression vs. depression) and so the authors have used columns to group the participants. The rows are the study variables.

A note on p values in descriptive tables

The *p*-value is a chi-square test used to help the reader determine if the differences across the columns are statistically significant or not. When you present a *p*-value in this way, think carefully about which test you want to use. A Pearson chi-square test will tell readers if the distribution of cell sizes differs significantly from what we would expect by chance. When your study variables have more than two categories however, it will not tell you if there is a linear trend across the categories. For example, if the outcome is no depression, moderate depression and severe depression, does the proportion of current smokers steadily increase as we move through these categories? Researchers would conduct a test for a linear trend in these circumstances.

It is useful to present data in this way because the readers can scan the table to identity that men with depression are significantly older, less educated, comprise more smokers and have more comorbidities. This helps characterise the data and also illustrate why it might be important to control for these variables in the main analysis. An alternative method favoured by many, is to show the *n*(%) in one of the categories (e.g. current smoker) rather than all of the categories (never, past, current). This saves space but still provides the important information. Most of the data are categorical, but for continuous variables (e.g. Charlson index, a measure of the expected burden of comorbidities), you should present the mean and standard deviation. Differences across the columns can be compared using a *t*-test.

Tables of descriptive statistics are followed by one or more tables that show results from the main analysis. It is quite common to first present a 'crude' estimate of relative risk, from a model that contains only the exposure of interest (here, depression). If the crude estimate is not sensible to report, for example, because it is heavily confounded by age and sex, then you may want to consider presenting a 'minimally adjusted' estimate (e.g. adjusting

Table 12.1 Baseline characteristics of 5411 men with valid 15-item Geriatric Depression Scale ratings, by depression status

	Group, percentage of participants		
Characteristic	No depression (n = 5072)	Depression (n = 339)	p value
Age group, in years			< 0.001
69–74	35.6	25.1	
75–79	43.1	44.2	
80–84	17.2	23.0	
>85	4.1	7.7	
Education			< 0.001
None	0.4	1.2	
Primary	15.1	24.5	
Some secondary	37.8	37.8	
Secondary	26.2	20.9	
Postsecondary	20.5	15.6	
Smoking			< 0.001
Never	33.2	20.4	
Past	61.8	70.4	
Current	5.0	9.2	
Duke Social Support Index tertile			< 0.001
Highest	44.7	9.0	
Middle	31.8	21.3	
Lowest	23.4	69.7	
Missing values	0.4	1.8	
Charlson index (weighted), mean (95% CI)	1.17 (1.12, 1.22)	2.21 (1.94, 2.48)	< 0.001
Missing values	11.3	4.1	

Source: [104]

for age and sex). Next, show the results adjusted for the proposed or possible confounding factors. This allows readers to see what happens to the association when the confounding factors are added to the model. This provides a sense of how biased the crude or minimally adjusted association might have been, had the confounders been ignored. Some authors present several sets of adjustments, perhaps adding additional confounders to the model, or perhaps showing separate models which contain different variables. In Table 12.2 the authors have also shown the association between the confounding factors and the outcome, which is something you might want to consider doing. It does

Table 12.2 Example table showing the association between confounding factors and outcome before and after adjustment for covariates

	Mean length of stay IRR (95% CI)		Total length of stay IRR (95% CI)		No. of hospital admissions IRR (95% CI)	
	Univariate	Multi-variate	Univariate	Multi-variate	Univariate	Multi-variate
Depression	1.32 (1.13,1.53)	1.25 (1.06,1.48)	1.76 (1.47,2.12)	1.65 (1.36,2.01)	1.30 (1.15,1.47)	1.22 (1.07,1.39)
Age		1.16 (1.10,1.23)		1.27 (1.18,1.36)		1.07 (1.02,1.13)
Education level		0.99 (0.94,1.04)		0.96 (0.91,1.02)		0.96 (0.92,1.01)
Duke Social Support Index tertiles		0.98 (0.92,1.04)		1.01 (0.94,1.09)		1.01 (0.96,1.07)
Smoking		0.94 (0.84,1.07)		0.82 (0.72,0.94)		0.88 (0.80,0.98)
Charlson index (weighted)		1.02 (0.99,1.04)		1.08 (1.05,1.11)		1.05 (1.03,1.07)

IRR = Incidence rate ratio

take up additional space, which is why many authors would only present the measure of relative risk for the exposure. Nonetheless, here we are able to see that other variables have an association with the outcome (chiefly age and Charlson index score) which is quite interesting.

Discussion

Having presented your results, it is now time to move on the discussion section. The discussion section is where you reflect on what was found, consider how the research questions were answered, summarise the strengths and limitations of your study, and appraise your study in light of the existing literature. A good discussion section is well-structured, and will allow non-technical readers to understand what you did, even if they did not understand your results section. Whereas the introduction section begins broad and ends with a narrow research question (imagine a funnel shape), the discussion section does the opposite. The discussion begins with a succinct summary of what was found, and then gradually broadens out to consider the wider implications of the study. Several commentators have proposed that discussion sections should have a tight structure, perhaps even with subheadings. Although many journals do not use subheadings in the discussion section, you may find it helpful to write the different parts of your discussion under these headings, each of which we will now consider.

Restate the main findings

In one or two sentences, tell the reader your 'bottom line' results. What did you find? Avoid simply repeating material from the results section. Imagine that you have only two sentences to describe the most important conclusions that can be drawn from your study. The discussion section is often written in plain English, rather than scientific or statistical language. For this reason, many readers, particularly journalists, might skip your methods and results sections entirely. They might go straight to your discussion section, and so you must grab their attention quickly but without over-simplifying things.

Strengths and limitations of the study

Every study has both strengths and limitations, and so does your study. Think of this section as a place where you can critically appraise your *own* research. It is important to show the readers that you are aware of the methodological and other shortcomings of what you did. When you have spent a long time conducting a piece of research, perhaps a year or perhaps even longer, it is tempting to think that your study has fewer limitations than it actually does. It is often said that that every mother thinks her baby is the most beautiful. Researchers can suffer from the same bias, often having a biased view about their work. Stand back from the research and imagine yourself to be a critical reviewer or reader. Was the research question really that important? Does the sample truly reflect the intended population? Was the exposure measured without bias? Was the statistical test used in fact the right one? Do the conclusions stay within the confines of the data? Really? When describing the strengths and limitations of your study, keep things balanced. Some limitations are widespread and readers will be sympathetic. Generally, we all have to rely on self-reports in questionnaires at some point, even if we would rather have available a gold standard. If the measures you used were reliable and validated, do not dwell too much on the well-known limitations of self-report. If you have conducted a trial, loss to follow-up is not a major flaw, unless it is severe and those dropping out were different kinds of people. Focus on the limitations which are more specific to your study. Before writing this section, have a look at other researchers' papers in academic journals. This will give you a sense of what kinds of issues should be discussed here.

Strengths and limitations in relation to other studies

In this section, start to make connections back to your introduction section, which would have briefly summarised the existing literature and identified important gaps in it. Compare your study with previous studies in the area, particularly more recent or more important ones, allowing readers to think about where your study 'fits' in the wider literature. Was your study bigger, better, more powerful *and* more useful than all previous studies? Probably not. Do not try to over-sell your paper – people will not buy it. Other studies may have had strengths which yours did not, although you may have moved the field forward by improving on key aspects. Explain how what you did was different, particularly emphasising any improvements on prior work. Do not get personal in this section. Focus on the research, not on the people who did it! If there are any important differences in the results, make sure you identify possible reasons for this. Was your population different in some important way? Did you measure the outcome differently? Finally, it should go without saying that it is much easier to write this section if you are familiar with the literature. This is another reason why it is so important to conduct a literature review prior to starting a research project. Remember that the literature may have changed since you did your literature review. It takes time to do research, and so new papers are likely to have been published since you began your project, particularly if your topic is popular, fast-moving or 'crowded' (meaning that many researchers are working in the same area). Return to the databases before you write up your results, to identity new studies. The last thing you want to do is claim that you were the first to find X, when in fact someone else published a paper finding X just last month!

Meaning of the study

The results are one thing, but what they mean is another. People critically appraising your research should be asking 'so what'? Too many research studies are published with little regard for their practical importance or reflection on how they move health sciences forward. For health sciences which are more theoretical in nature, such as health psychology, this section is where you need to say what your findings mean in terms of theory. Do your findings mean that the theory is supported, that it needs to be modified, or that it is simply wrong? For more data-focused disciplines, this section will tend to focus on practical implications. If you evaluated an intervention and it improved your outcome measure better than in a control group, then the meaning is fairly clear – it works. However, take great care to distinguish statistical from practical or clinical significance. Finding a statistically significant effect is one thing, but if the effect size is very small this might not be meaningful (in fact, it may be meaningless). Depending on the focus of your study, you might want to mention any economic implications of your results here. Health economists are interested in how much an intervention costs, in terms of the number of quality adjusted life years (QALYs) or other ways in which health can be measured. The impact of removing an exposure on population health might also be useful for readers. If you found that reducing coffee consumption would reduce the risk of having migraines for example, what are the public health benefits if people stop or reduce coffee consumption? How many people would it affect? For more applied health sciences, such as nursing or occupational therapy, in this section you should focus on what readers should do differently in their work. Based on your findings, should they continue doing what they always do, or do something differently?

Next steps and future

The final section of your discussion section should think ahead to the future. End your discussion as broadly as you opened your introduction section. Think about the wider field and the larger, ultimate implications. Avoid the temptation to become grandiose, and also avoid stepping beyond what you have actually found. Do, however, remind readers why the topic is important. They may have gotten lost in your results section and forgotten why the research question was worth asking at all. In the health sciences, different disciplines often share the same ultimate aims, so some of these statements make similar references (health improvement, population health, removing health inequalities, reducing costs of healthcare etc.). Each does an excellent job of making a final statement which should leave a lasting impression on the reader.

It is worth noting that someone skim-reading your paper, perhaps a journalist, might only look at the opening and closing sentences of your discussion section (assuming they get beyond the abstract). Make sure that these sentences count.

Co-authorship

It is important that all people who contributed to the manuscript are named as co-authors on the paper. Deciding who should be a co-author, and in what order they should be listed, is ideally done in advance of writing the paper. Disagreements can arise, and often do arise, at various stages of the writing process, including after publication. To avoid conflict, it is better to agree who the co-authors are before you start writing. If you are a student, do not assume that because the manuscript is from your project, you have sole claim as author. You are drawing on the contributions made by others, including your supervisor. Here are some of the people you might want to consider naming as a co-author:

- people who have made a substantive contribution to a study in other ways;
- study conception (i.e. the person who first had the idea to conduct the study);
- study design;
- data collection, analysis and interpretation;
- drafting the article and revising it (but not minor copy-editing).

If in doubt, seek advice from your supervisor. If you are taking the lead on writing up your results for publication, then you should be named as first author. If you decide not to write up your results however, your supervisor may write them up themselves. Do not forget that supervisors often make a substantial contribution to your work.

References

The reference list should be shown at the end of the article, usually before the figures and tables. In a dissertation, the reference list is likely to be quite long, because you need to cite all your sources. In a paper, journals often have limits on the number of references that you can include (e.g. 30 or 40). For this reason, you need to be selective and only cite references where you need to show the source of an idea, method or previous set of results.

Different journals have different guidelines for how reference lists should be presented. Software is available to help you format your reference list appropriately (e.g. EndNote or Reference Manager). You can also format yourself by hand, but this can be time-consuming, particularly if the journal asks for a numbered sequence of references. If you want to insert a new reference, you have to change the order of all subsequent numbers.

References are useful for people who read your research, because they can find out the source of the material for themselves. Similarly, when you read others' research, you will often follow-up their references in order to learn more. Referencing helps leave a 'trail of breadcrumbs' for other people, helping them navigate their way through the literature.

Plagiarism

Plagiarism is defined as the 'failure to credit sources of information used for an essay, report, project, journal article or book' (www.ucl.ac.uk/current-students/guidelines/plagiarism). Any contribution from others should be explicitly acknowledged as such (e.g. by naming co-authors). Given that most research builds on previous research, the contribution of other researchers is acknowledged by referencing their work. Great care must be taken to avoid taking other people's work and presenting this as your own. Good note keeping can help avoid situations in which you cannot remember the source of an idea or method. When quoting directly (e.g. three or more words), put the quotation in inverted commas to acknowledge that you are taking the exact words from a source.

The following are all examples of plagiarism:

- several quotations from different sources are combined together without identifying their sources;

- another person's ideas or theories are summarised without reference to that person in the text;

- a quotation is reproduced exactly, and without quotation marks (inverted commas);

- an idea expressed in a grant application to do a specific piece of research for the first time, is used by co-applicants who each publishes a paper stating that they are the first to do the same idea.

Check your institution's policy on plagiarism, and also the policy of any journal or publisher you intend to submit your work to. Policies may vary, but as a general rule, reference anything that isn't purely your own original idea. Even following this rule can lead to problems, if for example, you forget that you had read an idea somewhere and then subsequently believe that you generated the idea. The term 'implicit memory' is often invoked to explain why some academics appear to have absorbed an idea but forgot that they read it somewhere. Be careful, and keep detailed notes when you conduct literature reviews. Use reference management software, social bookmarking (e.g. CiteULike) and any tool that helps you keep track of your sources.

Conflicts of interest on other papers and grant applications

Conflicts of interest, or situations which be perceived as possible conflicts of interest, should either be avoided, or be declared. It is not wrong to have conflicts of interest, but trouble can arise when these interests might influence the publication process. Here are some examples of situations that may be considered conflicts of interest:

- Your line manager is a co-applicant on your grant application, but is writing a paper with someone else on the same topic, but he forgets to tell you.

- One of your co-authors is funded by the tobacco industry.

- You are paid to write an article about psychotropic medication for children with mood disorders, by a pharmaceutical company. The company says you cannot publish your article unless you the results are significant.

In the first example, your line manager should avoid this situation by declaring a possible conflict of interest and then withdrawing from your grant application. In the second example, it is not clear how to proceed. The fact that your co-author has received funding from the tobacco industry may not influence the results, but it may be perceived as having the potential to influence the results. In any case, this funding must be declared to the journal and publisher. In the third example, this is a clear conflict of interest. As an academic, you are entitled to freedom of expression. A funding body or other funding source should not have any influence over the analysis of results or of literature, nor the decision to publish. This situation should be avoided. If you are paid to write an article, you should be clear from the outset that you will publish regardless of the conclusions drawn. You should also declare that you were paid to write the article, even if you think the funder had no influence over your work.

If in doubt about whether you have a possible conflict of interest, it is better to make a declaration than not. Most journals will ask you to make a declaration when you submit a manuscript. Answers all questions honestly, and keep a detailed record of all declarations made. Many possible conflicts of interest are non-financial in nature. Conflicts of interest cannot be avoided all the time, there are often 'secondary' influences (e.g. personal rivalry, commitment to an institution, preference for a particular theory) which can influence decisions made in the research process. These are sometimes called 'dual commitments' or 'competing loyalties'. The important question is, how are you going to manage your conflicts of interest when they arise?

Choosing a journal

It is sometimes difficult to decide which journal is suitable to submit your paper to. You need to balance the impact factor of the journal, with the appropriate 'fit' to your paper. Impact factors are calculated based on the average number of times an article is cited during a specified time period (e.g. two years). Higher-impact health journals tend to be aimed at clinicians (e.g. *Lancet*, *BMJ*, *JAMA*). Lower-impact papers tend to be aimed at specific disciplines (e.g. *JAMA Dermatology*), or multidisciplinary readers (e.g. *Social Psychiatry* and *Psychiatric Epidemiology*). You can look at impact factors for various journals on their websites (also see impactfactor.weebly.com). One strategy is to look at your own reference list – what journals do you seem to be using? If several of your references are to papers published in *Social Science and Medicine*, then perhaps you should consider submitting your work there.

A tool called JANE (Journal/Author Name Estimator) can automatically search your abstract and generate a list of possible journals. To try it, go to http://www.biosemantics.org/jane.

Copy and paste your abstract into the box, then click on 'Find journals'. An example is shown below, using an abstract from a paper that was, in the end, submitted to the BMJ Open.

The top three suggestions, based on the content of the abstract, were *Journal of Homosexuality*, *BMC Public Health*, and *Archives of Pediatrics & Adolescent Medicine*.

When considering suggestions based on your abstract, as mentioned above, you need to think about the impact factor of the journal, not just the 'best fit' to your content. Both are important issues, and it can be difficult to get the balance right.

The manuscript submission process

Most manuscripts are submitted online, through a journal's online submission portal. Manuscript submission websites are often very similar to each other, but the requirements and attachments requested often vary. For example, to submit a paper to the *BMJ Open*, we would go to http://mc.manuscriptcentral.com/bmjopen. After logging in, we click on 'Author Centre' to submit a manuscript ('Reviewer Centre' is for when you have been asked to review someone else's manuscript).

You are taken through a series of pages, each prompting you to provide information about the manuscript you are submitting. For example, the first page asks for the article type, title, short title, and abstract. After this page,

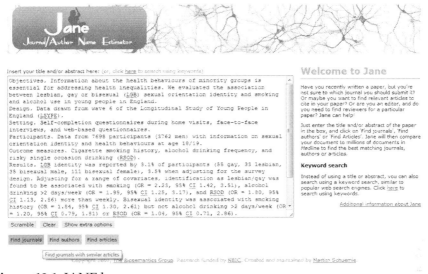

Figure 12.1 JANE home page

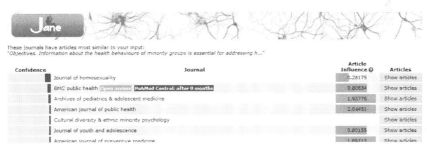

Figure 12.2 JANE suggestions page

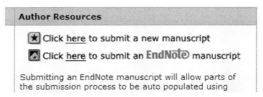

Figure 12.3 Accessing submissions page

you are asked for attributes about the manuscript, who the co-authors are, which peer reviewers you would prefer, any comments, the Word files containing your manuscript, and finally, you are asked to review a PDF of your manuscript generated by the website submission system. When you approve the manuscript PDF, it is sent to the editorial office for checking.

In conclusion, there is a variety of ways of disseminating your results. The majority of researchers however, focus on peer-reviewed journal articles. Journals are ranked according to impact factor, but this does not necessarily

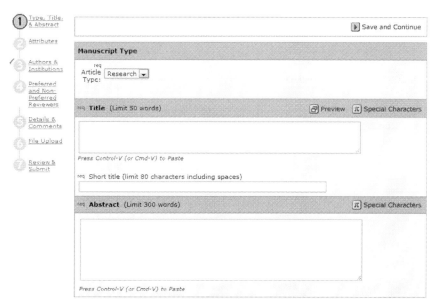

Figure 12.4 Submission description page

mean that a high-impact journal is always the best home for your research. When preparing a paper, you should reflect on publication ethics and think about who should be acknowledged – either as a co-author, in the reference list, or perhaps simply as an acknowledgement note. Learning how to write scientifically takes time, but we have a responsibility to take that time, because all results should eventually be published. Avoid the temptation to focus only on significant and important results. There is an ethical argument that researchers should always publish their work, regardless of the impact factor they would like aim for.

Linear regression for continuous outcomes

In previous chapters we have considered statistical models that contain only one exposure and a continuous outcome. *T*-tests and one-way ANOVA are examples of models that contain only one exposure. Typically this indicates whether people were exposed or unexposed, including where the exposure is a treatment condition in an experiment, compared to the control condition. We have learned that in observational studies, where confounding factors can distort the association between an exposure and an outcome, we may have to adjust for the confounder. In simple confounding scenarios this is relatively straightforward, using the stratification method introduced in Chapter 6. In reality, there are often several possible confounders and it is not straightforward to adjust by confounding by stratification. In this chapter, multiple linear regression is introduced as a method for adjusting for one or more confounding factors. The chapter starts by introducing simple linear regression before we add additional variables to the model.

Intended learning outcomes

By the end of this chapter, you should be able to:

- interpret the equation for linear regression;
- calculate the intercept and slope for a line of best fit;
- interpret regression coefficients;
- run multiple regression with more than one predictor variable;
- use categorical and dummy coded predictor variables;
- evaluate assumptions made by linear regression;
- transform predictor and outcome variables;
- understand standardised regression coefficients.

Introducing key terms

The term 'regression' originates from Francis Galton's observation that taller fathers tend to have shorter sons, and shorter sons tend to have taller fathers. This is because an extremely high or low measurement is likely to be followed by a less extreme value, closer to the mean than to the original measure. Values are said to 'regress' to the mean. Galton used regression equations to regress a set of observations on another set of observations, observing the tendency for the highest and lowest values to drift towards the average. Regression to the mean occurs in many different situations. A very good day at the stock market is likely to be followed by a more average day, rather than another very good day. An extremely hot week of weather is likely to be followed by a cooler spell, than another unusually hot week. The worst performing hospital one year is likely to improve the following year – it cannot 'move' to a worse position in a league table and so moves closer to the mean. Regression to the mean can be problematic when working with longitudinal data, for this reason. We are often unsure whether a change over time represents a real change, or the tendency for those with extreme values to move closer to the mean on the next measurement occasion. Most of the examples in this chapter treat observations as cross-sectional. The analysis of change using more complex regression models is beyond the scope of this book.

Regression models are widely used in the health sciences. When the outcome variable of interest is continuous, linear regression models are appropriate. When the outcome variable is categorical, logistic regression (discussed in the next chapter) is appropriate. If the outcome is time to event data, such as in survival analysis, then Cox regression is typically used (Chapter 9). Regression models are actually a family of models called generalised linear models, and they include t-test and ANOVA. As discussed below, ANOVA is actually a special case of linear regression when the predictor variables are categorical, and running the same analysis as regression will produce the same results as ANOVA. A good understanding of linear regression is necessary when conducting quantitative health research, and for interpreting the results of other people's studies.

The linear regression equation

The linear regression equation is used to create a statistical model that best predicts y (the dependent variable, or outcome) from x (the predictor variable, or exposure). The model is called a regression model. The linear regression equation is the equation of a straight line that best describes how y increases or decreases with each increase in the level of x. This is achieved using the method of least squares, described below. In practice, linear regression equations are usually obtained using statistical software. In this chapter, we will use the lm function in R to run linear regression models.

$$y = \beta_0 + \beta_1 x + e$$

The beta symbols refer to the parameters of the regression equation, and are often called 'beta coefficients'.

- y is the predicted value of the outcome

- x is the value of the predictor variable

- β_0 is the intercept parameter, which represents the estimated value of y when $x = 0$

- β_1 is the slope parameter, which represents the increase in y for every unit increase in x

- e represents the residual (error)

There are several assumptions made by the regression model, which are covered in more detail below.

The method of least squares

We need to find the parameter values for β_0 and β_1 that minimise the sum of the squared vertical distances between the data points and the regression line (line of best fit). We do this by estimating them, from these two formulae:

$$\beta_1 = \frac{\sum (x - \bar{x})(y - \bar{y})}{\sum (x - \bar{x})^2}$$

$$\beta_0 = \bar{y} - \beta_1 \bar{x}$$

To illustrate, Table 13.2 shows data from ten women who provided data on their waist measurement and on their age.

Linear regression in R

In the code below, we use the R function lm (linear model) to run a simple linear regression of waist (cm) on age at recruitment into the study at 1991. The dependent variable (waist) is regressed on the independent variable (age) as indicated by the tilde symbol (~). The model is given a name (lm1) and then we can type lm1 to obtain the results. Next, we can ask for a scatterplot showing the bivariate relationship between age and waist measurement. Finally, we fit the line of best fit from the regression model, onto the scatterplot.

Table 13.1 Example data for calculating least squares

Age	Waist	$(x-\bar{x})$	$(y-\bar{y})$	$(x-\bar{x})(y-\bar{y})$	$(x-\bar{x})^2$	$(y-\bar{y})^2$
56	87.00	1	6.368	6.37	1	40.5514
55	72.50	0	–8.132	0.00	0	66.1294
64	81.28	9	0.648	5.83	81	0.4199
69	76.20	14	–4.432	–62.05	196	19.6426
52	99.44	–3	18.808	–56.42	9	353.7409
46	88.90	–9	8.268	–74.41	81	68.3598
42	63.50	–13	–17.132	222.72	169	293.5054
63	90.81	8	10.178	81.42	64	103.5917
63	73.03	8	–7.602	–60.82	64	57.7904
40	73.66	–15	–6.972	104.58	225	48.6088
			SUM:	167.22	890	1052.3404

$\bar{x} = 55.00$ $\bar{y} = 80.632$

$\sum(x-\bar{x})(y-\bar{y})$	167.22
$\sum(x-\bar{x})^2$	890.00
β_1	0.19
β_0	70.30

Box 13.1 R code for linear regression

For the ten women in Table 13.1:

```
data <- read.table('age-waist.csv', header=TRUE, sep=',')
attach(data)
example <- lm(waist ~ age)
example
# We obtain an intercept coefficient of 70.2982 and a
# coefficient for age of 0.1879. This shows that the lm
# package in R produces the same results as when working by
# hand.
summary(lm)
```

For the larger data set (UK Women's Cohort Study):

```
data <- read.table('H:/My Documents/Book/Health sciences/
Worksheets/ukwcs_regression.csv', header=TRUE, sep=',')
attach(data)
lm1 <- lm(waist_2010 ~ age1991)
lm1
```

```
plot(age1991,waist_2010,main='Regression line predicting
waist measurements from age',xlab='Age in years',ylab='Waist
(cm)')
abline(lm1)
summary(lm1) #asks for the full output
```

The function abline adds the regression line to the scatterplot. This is a useful visual representation of the regression model. In the section below, we will think about what the regression coefficients mean.

What do the regression coefficients mean?

The intercept

The intercept refers to the point at which the regression line intercepts (crosses) the y-axis, and is the expected value of y when x is zero. The β_0 intercept of 98.32 therefore refers to the expected waist measurement when age is zero. This is not a meaningful value here, for two reasons. First, we should avoid using regression equations to predict values of y beyond that which are provided by the data. The available age range was 35 to 72 and so it could be very misleading to attempt to predict waist values below 35 or above 72. No data were available in the sample for these ages. Second, waist measurements at birth will not be this large. The association between age and waist is not linear across the life course, and so a different set of data with a different set of regression equations would be needed to predict values of waist in childhood and early adulthood. Our regression line only describes the linear relationship between age and waist between age 35 and 72. One way to make the intercept more meaningful is to 'centre' the predictor variable at its mean, described below. Although the intercept is often not useful, it is a necessary part of the regression equation. It provides the location/height of the regression line (see Figure 13.1).

The slope

The β_1 coefficient of –0.3769 refers to the expected change in waist measurement with each additional unit increase in age. Therefore, as age increases by one year, estimated waist measurement is expected to decrease by 0.38 cm. This coefficient provides the slope of the regression line.

Interpreting the output

The first part of the output simply reminds us that we have 'called' the lm function and shows us the model we requested (the regression of waist in 2010 on age in 1991). Next, the residuals are described. The smallest is –28.01, meaning that for one participant, the observed waist value was 28cm lower than the regression line. The largest residual is 41.87, meaning that for one

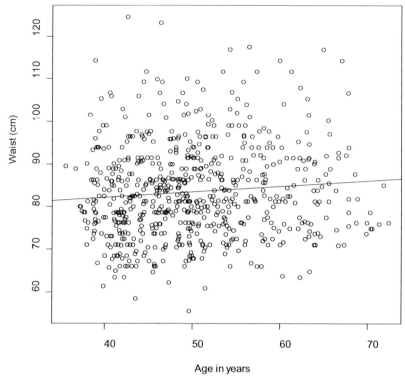

Figure 13.1 Regression line predicting waist measurements from age

```
Call:
lm(formula = waist_2010 ~ age1991)

Residuals:
    Min      1Q  Median      3Q     Max
-28.010  -8.073  -1.503   6.617  41.868

Coefficients:
            Estimate Std. Error t value Pr(>|t|)
(Intercept) 77.00919    2.71215  28.394  <2e-16 ***
age1991      0.13095    0.05353   2.446  0.0147 *
---
Signif. codes:  0 '***' 0.001 '**' 0.01 '*' 0.05 '.' 0.1 ' ' 1

Residual standard error: 10.9 on 665 degrees of freedom
Multiple R-squared: 0.00892,    Adjusted R-squared: 0.00743
F-statistic: 5.985 on 1 and 665 DF,  p-value: 0.01468
```

Figure 13.2 R output for linear regression

participant, the observed waist value was 42cm higher than the regression line. The median residual was –1.50 showing that the regression line ran fairly centrally through the data points. The first and third quartiles are also shown.

Next, the regression coefficients are shown. The intercept is estimated at 77.01 and this is the expected value of waist when age in 1991=0. The standard error is 2.61 and the t-statistic is provided. The p-value is statistically significant at $p < 0.001$, as indicated by the three asterisks. Of more interest is the coefficient for age in 1991, which is 0.13. This shows for each increase in age (in years), waist is predicted to increase by 0.13cm. This is statistically significant at $p < 0.05$ as indicated by the single asterisk. We can also obtain 95 per cent confidence intervals for the regression coefficients, by multiplying the standard error by 1.96 and either subtracting/adding this to/from the coefficient to obtain the lower/upper interval around the estimate. The standard error of the residuals refers to the average deviation of each y value around the estimated y values by the regression line. It is calculated by taking the square root of the sum of squared error and dividing this by the degrees of freedom.

Box 13.2 R code showing residuals from a simple linear regression model

```
data <- read.table('age-waist.csv', header=TRUE, sep=',')
attach(data)
example <- lm(waist ~ age)
plot(age,waist,main='Regression line predicting waist
measurements from age',xlab='Age in years',ylab='Waist
(cm)',type="n")
text(age,waist, labels=id)
abline(example)
points(age,fitted(example), pch=18, col="blue")
segments(age,waist,age,fitted(example),col="pink")
residuals(example)->lm.res; lm.res
```

The F-statistic and equivalence to ANOVA

The total variation in the outcome variable can be described using the total sum of squares. The variation described by the regression model can be described using the regression sum of squares. If we subtract the regression sum of squares from the total sum of squares, this provides the residual sum of squares, which is the sum of the squared deviations from the regression line. The partitioning of the variation in the outcome into two parts can be shown in an analysis of variance table.

If the regression line was a poor model of the association between x and y, the regression sum of squares would be similar to the residual sum of squares. An F-test can be used to test this (d.f. $= n-2$), using exactly the same method as described in Chapter 5. F- and t-tests are equivalent to linear regressions,

Table 13.2 Sources of variation in a linear regression

Source of variation	Sum of squares (SS)	d.f.	MS	F	R-squared
Regression	31.4186	1	31.4186	0.2462	0.0299
Residual	1020.9218	8	127.6152		
Total	1052.3404	9			

and you get exactly the same results if you run a *t*-test or ANOVA as a linear regression model.

$$SS_{total} = \sum (y - \bar{y}) = 1052.3404 \quad \text{(this value can be found in Table 13.1)}$$

$$SS_{regression} = \left[\sum (y - \bar{y})(x - \bar{x}) \right]^2 \Big/ \sum (x - \bar{x})^2 = 167.22^2 / 890 = 31.4186$$

The degrees of freedom are 1 for the regression sum of squares, and $n-2$ (= 8) for the residual sum of squares (total = 9).

R-squared and adjusted *R*-squared refer to the proportion of variance in *y* that is accounted for by the predictor variable. This statistic is more useful in multiple regression and is therefore discussed below.

Standardising predictor variables

Some predictor variables are not measured with meaningful units. For example, many psychosocial variables (e.g. quality of life, personality traits, mood) are self-reported on numerical scales where the meaning of the units is not clear. Similarly, a test of cognitive function might provide a score ranging from 5 to 50, but what does 1 point represent and how does this compare with another test of cognitive function? One solution is to standardise the scale, by subtracting the mean and dividing by the standard deviation of the variable. This produces a new variable, with a mean of 0 and a standard deviation of 1 (also called a z-score). One unit increase on this new scale refers to a one standard deviation increase, rather than a one unit increase. This can be helpful when comparing scales without meaningful units, with each other. A one standard deviation increase on a cognitive test can be compared to a one standard deviation increase on another test. Without knowing much about a test, it is useful to know what a 1 SD better score would be produce a one unit change in the *y* variable. Researchers also use standardised regression coefficients in a similar way to compare predictor variables and the outcome variable in terms of standard deviation change (described below).

Regression using centred age

It is often not sensible to use a regression model that refers to values outside the range of *x* or *y* available in the data. The intercept refers to the predicted waist at age 0 (i.e. birth) but our data did not contain any women at this age. Sometimes it is helpful to change the model so that the intercept refers to the mean age, rather than age 0. We can achieve this by first 'centring' age and then using centred age in the model, instead of actual age. Centring is achieved by subtracting the mean age from every value of age.

Box 13.3 R code for regression using centred age

```
data <- read.table('ukwcs_regression.csv', header=TRUE,
sep=',')
attach(data)
age_c=age1991-mean(age1991)
lm1 <- lm(waist_2010 ~ age_c)
lm1
plot(age_c,waist_2010,main='Regression line predicting waist
measurements from age',xlab='Age (centered)',ylab='Waist
(cm)')
abline(lm1)
summary(lm1)
```

As you can see from Figure 13.3, the regression line has exactly the same slope, but the interpretation of the intercept has changed. It is now the estimated waist value for someone with mean age, rather than age zero.

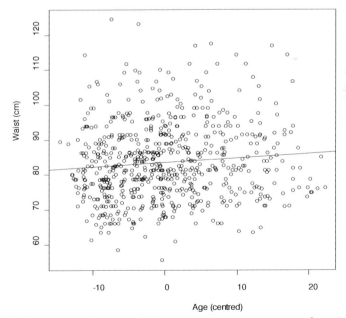

Figure 13.3 Regression line predicting waist measurements from age using centred age

Multiple linear regression

The x variable does not perfectly predict the y variable because the residual is not zero. There are probably other variables which predict y and the fact that we have a lot of residual variation is a clue that we might want to consider more than one (multiple) predictor variables to try and improve our predictive model and reduce the size of the residuals.

The residual + mean is the value of y if all the participants had the same x value. That is, the value of y controlling for x. Other terms are used synonymously with controlling for, such as conditioning on, residualising, partialling out, holding constant.

Educational attainment might also predict waist measurement, because we know from previous research that women with lower levels of educational attainment tend to have higher body mass index and waist measurements. In the data set, educational attainment is coded as a semi-continuous variable (0 = no qualifications, 1 = 'O' level, 2 = 'A' level, 3 = 'university degree'). We can use this variable as a continuous predictor variable. Strictly speaking, this variable is categorical or perhaps ordered categorical (ordinal). However, when there are several ordered categories researchers often treat such variables as continuous, since this is unlikely to cause too many problems. There are alternative approaches to handling semi-continuous and categorical predictor variables however, discussed below.

A strategy you might be tempted to try would be to conduct two linear regressions, one with age and one with educational attainment as the predictor variable. If we run these two models separately, we find that age explains 1per cent of the variance in waist measurements and educational attainment explains 2 per cent.

Box 13.4 R code for running two simple linear regression models separately

```
data <- read.table('ukwcs_regression.csv', header=TRUE,
sep=',')
attach(data)
lm1 <- lm(waist_2010 ~ age1991)
lm2 <- lm(waist_2010 ~ high_edu)
summary lm1
summary lm2
correlate(waist_2010,high_edu)
```

This does not mean however, that we have explained 1 + 2 = 3% of the variance. Age is negatively correlated with educational attainment (r = -0.23) indicating that younger women in the study had tended to reach higher levels of educational attainment. This means that variance in waist shared with age is also shared with educational attainment. We need to find a way to identify the unique contribution of age and educational attainment in predicting waist measurements, allowing or adjusting for the fact that these two predictor variables are correlated. Multiple regression is a good way to do this.

It might appear sensible to run a linear regression of waist on age first, and then use the residuals to perform another regression with educational attainment as the predictor. However, there is no particular reason why age should be given priority first, leaving educational attainment to predict whatever is left over. Multiple regression provides an estimate of the intercept and two slopes and calculates these simultaneously without giving priority to either variable. There are situations in which you might want to assume that one or more variables have priority over other variables, discussed below under hierarchical multiple linear regression, but for now we will focus on a simple example with two predictors having equal status.

Multiple regression is usually performed using statistical software rather than by hand. The equation for multiple regression with two independent variables however, is shown below.

$$y = \beta_0 + \beta_1 x_1 + \beta_2 x_2 + e$$

There is still one intercept, but there is a separate regression coefficient for each predictor variable. Effectively, this equation is estimating a three-dimensional 'plane' of best fit, rather than a line of best fit. It may be helpful to visualise a three-dimensional graph with three axes, x_1, x_2 and y. If we wanted to predict y, we would multiply each x variable by its regression coefficient and then add this to the intercept value.

Running a multiple regression in R

The code for multiple regression is very similar to simple regression, using a plus sign (+) to add additional predictor variables.

Box 13.5 R code for multiple regression with two predictor variables

```
lm3 <- lm(waist_2010 ~ age1991 + high_edu)
summary(lm3)
```

Interpreting the output

The interpretation of the intercept in the output from multiple regression is different to that from simple linear regression. It is the predicted value of waist when age is zero and when educational attainment is zero (81.24cm). The beta coefficients for the predictor variables are the expected change in the outcome variable per unit increase in the predictor variable, holding the other predictor variable constant. For example, as age increases by one year, we expect waist to increase by 0.09cm (holding education constant). As educational attainment increases by one level, we expect waist to decrease by –1.29cm (holding age constant). The coefficients differ from those obtained when running two

```
Call:
lm(formula = waist_2010 ~ age1991 + high_edu)

Residuals:
    Min      1Q  Median      3Q     Max
-27.806  -7.979  -1.489   6.857  40.518

Coefficients:
            Estimate Std. Error t value Pr(>|t|)
(Intercept) 81.23859    3.04561  26.674  < 2e-16 ***
age1991      0.09376    0.05465   1.716  0.08667 .
high_edu    -1.29364    0.43327  -2.986  0.00293 **
---
Signif. codes:  0 '***' 0.001 '**' 0.01 '*' 0.05 '.' 0.1 ' ' 1

Residual standard error: 10.84 on 664 degrees of freedom
Multiple R-squared: 0.02205,    Adjusted R-squared: 0.0191
F-statistic: 7.486 on 2 and 664 DF,  p-value: 0.0006097
```

Figure 13.4 R output for multiple regression

separate regressions, because this multiple regression allows for the fact that age and educational attainment are correlated.

Using regression coefficients from multiple regression to predict outcome variables

We can use the coefficients above to estimate values of our outcome variable using known values of our predictor variables. This is the ultimate aim of regression models – prediction. For example, suppose that a woman is 55 years old and has a university degree. What is her expected waist measurement value?

$$y = 81.2386 + (0.0938 \times 55) + (-1.2936 \times 3) = 82.52$$

Here, you can see that we 'insert' the known (observed) value of x_1 (age) and x_2 (educational attainment) into the regression equation, multiplying each coefficient by the known value. We predict a waist size of 82.52cm for this person. Note however, that overall the model explains rather little of the variance in waist measurements, so this may not be a particularly accurate prediction. Now suppose a woman is 80 years old and has no educational qualifications. What is her expected waist measurement value?

$$y = 81.2386 + (0.0938 \times 80) + (-1.2936 \times 0) = 88.74$$

The expected value this time is 88.74cm. Note that having no educational qualifications is coded 0 in the data, and when we multiply the coefficient for education by zero this equals zero.

Hierarchical multiple regression

Multiple regression models can be ordered sequentially, to evaluate whether the addition of new predictor variables improves the prediction capacity of the model. Here, we compare a 'basic' model containing only age, with three additional models: one with socio-economic status variables (educational and occupational social class), one which additionally controls for health behaviours (smoking, alcohol, fruit and vegetable intake) and one which additionally controls for self-rated health. These are labelled lm_basic, lm_ses, lm_hb, lm_full.

Box 13.6 R code for hierarchical multiple linear regression

```
lm_basic <- lm(waist_2010 ~ age1991)
lm_ses <- lm(waist_2010 ~ age1991 + high_edu + nssec_max)
lm_hb <- lm(waist_2010 ~ age1991 + high_edu + nssec_max +
smoker + drinker)
lm_full <- lm(waist_2010 ~ age1991 + high_edu + nssec_max +
smoker + drinker +healthy)
# We can compare the performance of models using the anova
# command.
anova(lm_basic,lm_ses)
anova(lm_ses,lm_hb)
anova(lm_hb,lm_full)
```

Interpreting the output

Comparing the basic model with the SES model (Figure 13.5), we can see that the SES model fits significantly better than the basic model ($p < 0.01$). Athough not shown in this figure, the health behaviours model however, does not fit significantly better than the SES model ($p = 0.92$), suggesting that these variables (smoking and alcohol drinking) add little to the prediction of waist measurements. Adding self-rated health however, significantly improves model fit ($p < 0.01$) suggesting that this is worth including.

```
> anova(lm_basic,lm_ses)
Analysis of Variance Table

Model 1: waist_2010 ~ age1991
Model 2: waist_2010 ~ age1991 + high_edu + nssec_max
  Res.Df    RSS Df Sum of Sq      F   Pr(>F)
1    665  79023
2    663  77847  2    1176.3 5.0092 0.006931 **
---
Signif. codes:  0 '***' 0.001 '**' 0.01 '*' 0.05 '.' 0.1 ' ' 1
> |
```

Figure 13.5 R output for hierarchical multiple linear regression

Categorical predictor variables

We may want to include categorical predictor variables (e.g. sex, smoker vs. non-smoker) in a regression model. This is quite straightforward when the categorical predictor has only two values (e.g. 0 or 1). These variables can be entered into the regression model in the same way as continuous variables. The interpretation of the coefficient is the change in the outcome variable as the categorical predictor changes from 0 to 1. For ordered categorical variables (e.g. a scale ranging from 1 to 5) the interpretation would assume a linear increase per unit increase on this scale. This assumes that the distance between 1 and 2 is the same as the distance between 2 and 3. Such an assumption may not be correct. Researchers, particularly in psychology, often treat ordered categorical variables with at least 5 and preferably 7 categorical as continuous. They assume that the scale represents some underlying variable which does have continuous properties. If you have a categorical variable where this assumption is questionable, you may want to consider creating categorical variables from the scale. To achieve this, we create dummy variables and use these in the regression model instead of the original scale. Dummy variables involve choosing a reference group (e.g. no educational qualifications) and then creating a new binary variable for all of the other variables, coded 1 for those who belong in that category and 0 for those who do not. In the case of the educational attainment variable, this results in three new dummy variables from the original four values on the scale:

- O level (vs. no qualifications)
- A level (vs. no qualifications)
- degree (vs. no qualifications)

These three variables are then entered into the regression, treated as binary variables in the usual way. A straightforward way to do this in R is to create a copy of the original scale, which we will call edu_cat, and then declare this to be a 'factor' variable (categorical variable). When edu_cat is entered into a regression model, R will create dummy variables automatically. In the example below, we will use the weight data and evaluate whether educational attainment categories predict waist, holding age constant.

> **Box 13.7** R code for transforming a continuous variable into a categorical variable
>
> ```
> attach(data) edu_cat <- factor(high_edu, labels =
> c("(none)","(O level)","(A level)","(Degree)"))
> lm_educat <- lm(waist_2010 ~ age1991 + edu_cat)
> summary(lm_educat)
> ```

```
Call:
lm(formula = waist_2010 ~ age1991 + edu_cat)

Residuals:
    Min      1Q  Median      3Q     Max
-27.537  -7.854  -1.304   7.029  40.905

Coefficients:
                   Estimate Std. Error t value Pr(>|t|)
(Intercept)        83.17064    3.42679  24.271  < 2e-16 ***
age1991             0.08847    0.05576   1.587  0.11310
edu_cat(O level)   -3.38699    1.62006  -2.091  0.03694 *
edu_cat(A level)   -4.52540    1.66800  -2.713  0.00684 **
edu_cat(Degree)    -5.29774    1.63777  -3.235  0.00128 **
---
Signif. codes:  0 '***' 0.001 '**' 0.01 '*' 0.05 '.' 0.1 ' ' 1

Residual standard error: 10.85 on 656 degrees of freedom
Multiple R-squared: 0.02682,    Adjusted R-squared: 0.02089
F-statistic:  4.52 on 4 and 656 DF,  p-value: 0.001313
```

Figure 13.6 R output using dummy variables

Interpreting the output

All three of the dummy variables show the estimated change in waist, for the educational category shown compared to the reference group (no educational qualifications). Women with O levels have estimated waist measurements 3.39cm lower than the reference group, with A levels 4.53cm lower, and with a degree 5.30cm lower. This is evidence for a dose-response association between educational attainment and waist measurement (as educational attainment increases, waist decreases). Such evidence could be used to support the conclusion that treating educational attainment as a continuous scale is justified – there is a clear graded linear relationship. Linearity should be tested rather than assumed however, so it is worth checking whether results differ when treating ordered categorical variables as categories compared to treating them as linear.

Adjusting for possible mediators to evaluate attenuation of an effect

We may be interested in a particular exposure x and its association with y, but also in possible mediators that explain the association between x and y. The concept of mediation was introduced in Chapter 6. One way to evaluate the explanatory role of possible mediators is to add them to a regression equation, one at a time, an equation that already contains the exposure of interest and key confounders such as age or sex. The percentage attenuation of the x–y association (available from the coefficient for x in the first model) when the proposed mediator is added (available from the coefficient for x in the second model, additionally containing the mediator) can be calculated using the formula below. This attenuation indicates by how much the mediator explains the association between x and y.

$$100 \times \left[\left(B_{model1} - B_{model2} \right) / B_{model1} \right]$$

As an example, suppose that we are interested in the association between number of cigarettes smoked and weight in female smokers. First, we will create a nested sample of smokers from a dataset that contains information on weight, smoking and diet. Next, we will calculate the association between number of cigarettes smoked and weight. Following that, we will additionally adjust for dietary quality (defined as eating five or more fruits or vegetables per day). Finally, we will consider another possible mediator, number of alcoholic drinks consumed, to see if this explains the association between cigarettes and weight.

```
dietdata <- read.table('ukwcs_regression_diet.csv',
header=TRUE, sep=',')
attach(dietdata)
(smokers <- dietdata [dietdata$smoker ==1, ]) #subsets the
# smokers, created a nested sample of smokers
attach(smokers) #attach the nested sample of smokers
lm_smokers <- lm(weight_kg2010 ~ age1991 + n_cigs)
summary(lm_smokers)
lm_smokers_diet <- lm(weight_kg2010 ~ age1991 + n_cigs +
gooddiet)
summary(lm_smokers_diet)
100*((0.2674-0.2564)/0.2674) #4.11% attenuation
```

Diet explains 4 per cent of the association between number of cigarettes smoked and weight. Now let's evaluate another possible mediator. Women who smoke more cigarettes might also engage in less physical activity and have poor diets, leading to higher waist measurements. Perhaps waist mediates the association between cigarettes and weight?

```
lm_smokers_waist <- lm(weight_kg2010 ~ age1991 + n_cigs +
waist_2010)
summary(lm_smokers_waist)
100*((0.2674-0.0389)/0.2674) #85.25% attenuation
```

Waist appears to explain 85 per cent of the association between smoking and weight. There are two important points to note about these results:

1 The status of the mediating variable should be guided by substantive knowledge about the variables, existing evidence, and theory. It may not be appropriate to assume that diet or waist measurements lie on a causal chain between cigarettes. This is particularly true for cross-sectional data. Ideally, mediators should be measured later in time than exposures

(they come after the exposure). Such longitudinal measurements are not always available, and so researchers frequently use theory to justify claiming that a variable might be a mediator. Health behaviours other than smoking might be confounding factors, rather than mediators.

2 Unlike hierarchical regression, where we add further variables to existing groups of variables, this 'effect decomposition' approach involves adding each proposed mediator separately to the basic model. Do not add mediators to existing models that already contain other mediators. Calculate the percentage attenuation for one proposed mediator at a time.

Adding interaction terms to evaluate effect modification

Effect modification was introduced in Chapter 6. In linear regression, effect modification is evaluated by adding an 'interaction term' between the exposure and the possible modifier. The interaction term is created by calculating the product of (multiplying) the exposure and the modifier. This term is entered into the regression model, along with the exposure and modifier.

```
attach(data)
lm_modifier <- lm(waist_2010 ~ age1991 + nssec_max +
age1991:nssec_max)
summary(lm_modifier)
```

The interaction term represents the combined effect of scoring one unit higher on both variables, after the unique effect of each variable has been held constant. It can also be described as the 'excess risk' due to interaction, if the combined effect of each variable increases the risk of a hazardous outcome. To identify significant effect modification, we can create a 'global' test of interaction for the whole model, comparing this to a nested model that does not contain the interaction term.

```
lm_basic<- lm(waist_2010 ~ age1991 + nssec_max)
summary(lm_ basic)
anova(lm_modifier,lm_basic)
```

Although the p value of 0.06 is not statistically significant at the $p < 0.05$ level, many commentators argue that values < 0.10 or even 0.20 warrant an exploration of possible effect modification. We could simply report the model coefficients including the interaction term, but this may be difficult for readers to interpret. One solution is to separate results by stratifying the modifier (age), in other words, creating age groups.

```
(professional <- data [data$nssec_max==1 ,]) #subsets
# professional women
```

```
attach(professional) #attach the nested sample of professional
# women
lm_professional<- lm(waist_2010 ~ age1991)
summary(lm_professional)
```

The coefficient for age in the professional group is 0.22, indicating a 0.22 increase in waist per year of age among this group.

```
(lower <- data [data$nssec_max==2 | nssec_max==3 ,]) #subsets
# lower than professional women (intermediate or manual)
attach(lower) #attach the nested sample of lower women
lm_lower<- lm(waist_2010 ~ age1991)
summary(lm_lower)
```

The coefficient for age in the intermediate and manual group is –0.01 and is not statistically significant, indicating that age is not a significant predictor of waist in this group. We can conclude that occupational social class appears to modify the association between age and waist: the association is specific to the professional group. Note however, that there may be confounding factors we have not considered, such as chronic disease and smoking.

R-squared

R-squared is the square of the correlation coefficient r, and is calculated as $SS_{regression}/SS_{total}$. It is the proportion of variance in y that has been explained by the regression model. Put differently, it tells us how much variation in y is accounted for by the set of x variables. A 'better' regression model will account for more variation in y, a less good model will account for less. As a set, age and educational attainment account for 2.2 per cent of the variance in waist measurements. This still leaves much variation unexplained, suggesting that we need to find additional predictors for our model.

Checking assumptions

These are some important assumptions made in multiple regression:

- absence of multicollinearity;
- the residuals (errors) are normally distributed;
- the variance of the residuals is consistent across y;
- the residuals are independent;
- no influential cases and outliers;
- no skewness and kurtosis in y

There are other assumptions made in regression models, but these three are arguably the most important. You should also consider outliers and influential cases, described below, because these can influence the model and the regression coefficients and therefore conclusions you might draw. In this section we will evaluate these assumptions using R for a basic regression model, predicting waist from age in the same sample of ten women used earlier. When evaluating your own data, modify the R code accordingly.

Box 13.8 R code for regression model 'example' used to illustrate checking of assumptions

```
data <- read.table('age_waist.csv', header=TRUE, sep=',')
attach(data)
example <- lm(waist ~ age)
```

Absence of multicollinearity

Multicollinearity can be evaluated by requesting a correlation matrix showing the bivariate correlation between each pair of variables. Look for high or perfect correlations, as this could indicate multicollinearity. It is relatively unusual to have multicollinear variables. Another example, which you could not check simply by looking at correlations, is if you had scores from four parts of a test, and then also the total score. You could not put the four scores and the total score in a regression model – the total score is a linear combination of the four scores. Multicollinearity can also be evaluated using variance inflation factor (VIF). In multiple linear regression, you can request VIF values when there are more than two variables, using the command vif(example) where example is the label for the regression model. Values above 10 are thought to indicate strong and therefore worrying linear relationships between each variable and other variables in the model. Consider dropping one or more of these additional variables in such a situation, focusing on the most substantively important variable instead. For example, you might want to include only the total score on a test rather than scores from separate parts of the test.

Normally distributed residuals

To check whether the residuals are normally distributed, use the R function hist(lm.res) to request a histogram. With the small sample size ($n = 10$) used in our example, we are unlikely to achieve a good normal distribution, but you can modify this code for your own data or try it on a larger data set. The functions qqnorm(lm.res) and qqline(lm.res) are used to request a normal Q-Q plot which is also useful for evaluating normality. Look for points along the straight line. A curvy S-shape can indicate non-normality of the residuals (see Figure 13.7: Panel C). The shapiro.qqnorm(lm.res,type="n") command available in the epicalc package provides a p-value comparing the distribution to an equivalent normal distribution having the same mean and standard deviation. If the p-value is non-significant, it indicates that our distribution is not significantly different from this normal distribution. Note, however, that in large sample sizes the Shapiro–Wilk test often produces significant p-values owing to small and often trivial non-normality. Arguably, although it is more subjective, a visual approach to evaluating non-normality using the Q-Q plot is more useful when working with large sample sizes.

Box 13.9 R code for evaluating the normality of residuals assumption

```
hist(lm.res) #The distribution of residuals, if the model
# fits well, should be normal
require(car)
qqPlot(example, main="QQ Plot")
```

The variance of the residuals consistent across Y

If this assumption is violated, the data are said to show heteroscedasticity. We do not want more variance at certain levels of y, and less variance at other levels of y. We can plot the predicted values against the residuals, to evaluate this assumption.

Box 13.10 R code for evaluating heteroscedasticity

```
require(car)
ncvTest(example)
spreadLevelPlot(example)
```

The residuals are independent

This means that there is no autocorrelation in the residuals, that is, one participant's residual is correlated with another participant's residual. This might occur for example, if the same participant has appeared twice in the data set, perhaps in error. It is important that each observation is unique and not from the same person. The Durbin–Watson test is used to evaluate independence of the residuals.

Box 13.11 R code for evaluating independence of the residuals

```
durbinWatsonTest(example)
```

Outliers and influential cases

An outlier is a case that might exert too much influence on the regression line, perhaps because it is an extreme value. For example, someone with an age of 110 is relatively unusual, and could bias the regression line by changing the intercept and the slope. Univariate outliers refer to extreme values on one variable. Multivariate outliers can also be problematic. These concern extreme combinations of two or more variables (e.g. consider someone with an age of 18, but a salary of £100,000. Both values are plausible when considered separately, but when considered together this person is probably a multivariate outlier). Univariate outliers can be identified using Cook's distance (see below). Multivariate outliers can be identified using Mahalanobis distance.

Box 13.12 R code for identifying influential cases

Values which are univariate outliers, multivariate outliers and values of the outcome variable which have a strong influence on the predictor variables (said to have high 'leverage') can be identified using the code below.

```
outlier_data <- read.table('age_waist_outlier.csv',
header=TRUE, sep=',')
attach(outlier_data)
outlier_example <- lm(waist ~ age)
plot(age,waist,main='Regression model (with outlier)',xlab='
Age',ylab='Waist (cm)')
abline(outlier_example)
summary(outlier_example)
require(car)
avPlots(outlier_example)
cutoff <- 4/((nrow(mtcars)-length(outlier_
example$coefficients)-2))
plot(outlier_example, which=4, cook.levels=cutoff) #Panel C
influencePlot(outlier_example, id.method="identify",
main="Influence Plot", sub="Circle size is propartial to
Cook's Distance" ) #Panel D
```

Figure 13.7 shows how an outlier (a women with an age of 90) can have a dramatic effect on the regression line. In Panel A, the regression line is flattened because this high value of age has a strong influence on the line of best fit. The coefficient for age is –0.0060. This implies a flat regression line and no association between age and waist. Removing this outlier results in a positive slope (B = 0.1879), and may better reflect the relationship between age and waist. It is important to note that an outlier can have a small residual, because the line of best fit will still take this person into account. Nonetheless, this participant's data has strong leverage (influence) on the regression line.

Skewness and kurtosis

Positive and negative skew were introduced in Chapter 1. When the distribution of a variable is negatively skewed, log transformation can be used to normalise the distribution. When a distribution is positively skewed, taking the square root of the variable can help normalise the distribution. Different

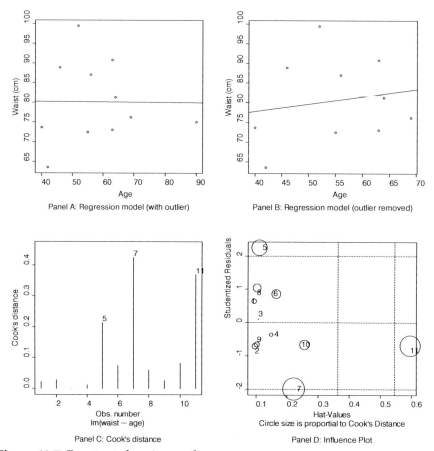

Figure 13.7 R output showing outliers

kinds of transformations, and the situations in which you might want to use them, are discussed in more detail below.

Box 13.13 R code for quick check of model assumptions

The following code can be used as a quick check for skewness, kurtosis and heteroscedasticity.

```
library(gvlma)
gvmodel <- gvlma(example)
summary(gvmodel)
```

Transforming variables

Log transformations

Negatively skewed distributions (skewed to the left) often occur. Reaction time is a good example of a variable that usually produces a negatively skewed distribution. We can measure people's reaction times, but some will be quite slow to respond, producing a long tail in the distribution. Log transformation of the variable can help address the problem. If the predictor is log transformed, then the coefficients still imply a linear change in y per increase in $\log x$.

Box 13.14 R code for linear regression with a log transformed predictor variable

```
rt_data <- read.table('ukwcs_regression_rt.csv',
header=TRUE, sep=',')
(rt_data2 <- rt_data [rt_data$srt_mean<1000, ]) #removes
# outliers above 1000m/s
attach(rt_data2) #attach the data with outliers removed
hist(srt_mean)
lnsrt<-log(srt_mean)
hist(lnsrt)
diet<-vegetables+fruit
diet_example <- lm(diet ~ age1991+nssec_max+lnsrt)
summary(diet_example)
```

The coefficient for log reaction time is −5.5167. This means that for each increase in log reaction time, diet decreases by 5.52 points. The interpretation of this coefficient is not straightforward, unless we work out the expected increase between two values on the original scale (milliseconds). For example, suppose we can estimate the difference in y between 750 milliseconds and 500 milliseconds reaction time. These two scores can be labelled r_1 and r_2 respectively. The formula below shows how to do this:

$$y = \beta_1 \times \left(\log(r_1) - \log(r_2) \right) = \beta_1 \times \log\left(\frac{r_1}{r_2} \right)$$
$$y = -5.5167 \times \log\left(\frac{750}{500} \right) = -5.5167 \times 0.4055 = -2.2370$$

This means that as reaction time increases from 500 to 750 milliseconds, the diet score decreases by 2.24 points. An alternative approach would be to express the increase in reaction time as a percentage. For example, to estimate the change in diet score for a 50 per cent increase in reaction time, use the log of 1.5 in the equation:

$$y = \beta_1 \times \log(1.5) = -2.2368$$

```
Call:
lm(formula = diet ~ age1991 + nssec_max + lnsrt)

Residuals:
    Min      1Q  Median      3Q     Max
-25.589  -9.977  -1.336   7.394  78.989

Coefficients:
             Estimate Std. Error t value Pr(>|t|)
(Intercept) 60.276986  14.442524   4.174 3.56e-05 ***
age1991      0.002081   0.090655   0.023   0.9817
nssec_max   -1.685476   0.793897  -2.123   0.0343 *
lnsrt       -5.516718   2.479323  -2.225   0.0265 *
---
Signif. codes:  0 '***' 0.001 '**' 0.01 '*' 0.05 '.' 0.1 ' ' 1

Residual standard error: 13.06 on 480 degrees of freedom
Multiple R-squared: 0.01961,    Adjusted R-squared: 0.01348
F-statistic: 3.201 on 3 and 480 DF,  p-value: 0.02315
```

Figure 13.8 R output for linear regression with a log-transformed predictor variable

This means that for a 50 per cent increase in reaction time, diet score decreases by 2.24 points.

Outcome variables with a preponderance of zeros

If your outcome variable has a preponderance of zeros there are several strategies available. For example, you could compare the zeros with other values, grouping the other values together, and then use logistic regression (see Chapter 14). Alternatively, you could use zero-inflated regression, which is beyond the scope of this book. You could also restrict the regression to people with non-zero values (e.g. only the smokers).

Non-normality in outcome variables

If an outcome variable in not normally distributed, you may want to transform it to normalise the distribution. As mentioned above, taking the natural logarithm of a positively skewed variable, for example, can normalise a distribution. The log transformed variable can be used as an outcome variable in linear regression.

If the outcome is log-transformed, the regression coefficient refers to the expected *log* change in y per unit increase in the x variable, holding other x variables constant. To obtain the one *unit* increase in y, you have to take the exponent of the coefficient exp(B). For example, using log reaction time as an outcome variable, the coefficient for age is 0.006812 in a simple linear regression model (see Box 13.15). This means for each year of age, reaction time increases by log(0. 006812) or 1.0068 milliseconds (the exponent of 0. 006812 is 1.006835254).

Predictor variables with a preponderance of zeros

Although predictor variables do not have to be normally distributed, there are some distributions that may require transformation. Number of cigarettes smoked, for example, has a preponderance of zeros because many people are non-smokers. We can create a new variable (smoker/non-smoker coded 1/0) and put this variable into the regression along with number of cigarettes smoked.

There are three models shown in this example:

1. including only smokers and controlling for number of cigarettes;

2. including all participants and controlling for number of cigarettes;

3. including all participants and controlling for smoking status and number of cigarettes.

Box 13.15 R code for linear regression with a natural log-transformed outcome variable

```
rt_data <- read.table('ukwcs_regression_rt.csv',
header=TRUE, sep=',')
attach(rt_data)
hist(srt_mean)
lnsrt<-log(srt_mean)
hist(lnsrt)
rt_example <- lm(lnsrt ~ age1991)
summary(rt_example)
```

Box 13.16 R code for linear regression of waist on number of cigarettes smoked per day, among smokers

```
rt_data <- read.table('ukwcs_regression_rt.csv',
header=TRUE, sep=',')
(smokers <- rt_data [rt_data$smoker ==1, ]) #subsets the
# smokers, created a nested sample of smokers
attach(smokers) #attach the nested sample of smokers
lm_example1 <- lm(waist_2010 ~ age1991 + n_cigs)
summary(lm_example1)
attach(rt_data)
lm(example2) <- lm(waist_2010 ~ age1991 + n_cigs)
summary(example2)
attach(rt_data)
lm_example3 <- lm(waist_2010 ~ age1991 + smoker + n_cigs)
summary(lm_example3)
```

```
Coefficients:
            Estimate Std. Error t value Pr(>|t|)
(Intercept)  66.0895     6.7363   9.811   <2e-16 ***
age1991       0.3113     0.1347   2.311   0.0221 *
n_cigs        0.2219     0.1046   2.121   0.0354 *
---
Signif. codes:  0 '***' 0.001 '**' 0.01 '*' 0.05 '.' 0.1 ' ' 1
```

Figure 13.9 R output for linear regression of waist on number of cigarettes smoked per day: example 1

In the first example, the coefficient of 0.2219 shows that among smokers and adjusted for age, each additional cigarette per day is associated with a 0.22 cm increase in waist measurement. The second example shows what would happen if we included both smokers and non-smokers in the regression model. The coefficient is reduced to 0.11 and is non-significant, probably because the model is incorrectly specified. In the second example, the dose-response association between number of cigarettes smoked and waist measurement is under-estimated.

In the third example, the coefficient of –2.17995 for smoking status means that for smokers, the waist measurement is 2.18cm lower than for non-smokers. However, the coefficient of 0.22081 means that controlling for smoking status, each cigarette is associated with a 0.2208cm increase in waist measurement. The regression coefficient for n_cigs is the linear effect among the exposed group of smokers. The regression coefficient for the smoker variable represents the difference between the non-smoking group and the extrapolated linear trend for the number of cigarettes when the number of cigarettes is zero. Put differently, smokers have waist measurements –2.18cm different than non-smokers if they theoretically smoked 0 cigarettes, –2.18 + 1 × (0.22) if they smoked 1 cigarette, –2.18 + 20 × (0.22) if they smoked 20, and so on. This method captures the distribution of cigarettes appropriately, allowing for the group of non-smokers and a linear trend (dose-response effect) among smokers, in the same model. Our results suggest that smokers have smaller waist measurements than non-smokers, but that heavier smokers tend to have larger waist measurements.

```
Coefficients:
            Estimate Std. Error t value Pr(>|t|)
(Intercept) 71.12288    3.52275  20.190  < 2e-16  ***
age1991      0.25279    0.07278   3.473 0.000561  ***
smoker      -2.17995    1.62941  -1.338 0.181573
n_cigs       0.22081    0.10546   2.094 0.036794  *
---
Signif. codes:  0 '***' 0.001 '**' 0.01 '*' 0.05 '.' 0.1 ' ' 1
```

Figure 13.10 R output for linear regression of waist on number of cigarettes smoked per day: example 2

258

Standardised regression coefficients

Standardised regression coefficients can often be useful in multiple regression, because they allow us to compare the effect sizes across variables measured on different scales. A standardised regression coefficient refers to the predicted standard deviation change in the outcome per standard deviation change in the predictor variable. One way to obtain them is to first standardise the predictor variables by subtracting the mean and dividing the standard deviation (as described above) and then run the regression model with these new variables. However, many statistical packages provide them automatically. To obtain standardised coefficients in R:

```
#The scale function creates a new version of the dataset with
# mean=0 and SD=1
data.std <- scale(data)
#This is converted from a matrix to a data frame
data.std <- as.data.frame(data.std)
#Check that the means are 0 and the SDs are 1
mean(data.std)
sd(data.std)
#Run the regression model again with the new dataset
data.mod.std <- lm(waist_2010 ~ age_c, data = data.std)
#This provides the standardised regression coefficients
summary(data.mod.std)
```

When there is one predictor variable, the standardised regression coefficient is equivalent to the Pearson correlation coefficient (r, which means 'regression'). In the regression context, x is thought to predict y, whereas in the correlation context we may not make a prediction about which variable predicts the other. Some researchers might refer to each as x_1 and x_2, for this reason. Statistically, both approaches produce the same value, and both simply summarise the variance shared by both variables.

Summary

In this chapter we have introduced simple and multiple linear regression, and explained that several other techniques (including ANOVA) are special cases of regression models. Regression modelling is central to many forms of data analysis and so it is worth learning about regression in order to analyse your data and interpret the results from published studies. In the next chapter, we will consider regression models where the outcome is categorical using logistic regression.

Further reading

Tabachnick B, Fidell L, *Using Multivariate Statistics*. Harlow: Pearson Education, 2007.

Logistic regression for categorical outcomes

If you want to model the association between an exposure/intervention and an outcome that is categorical, then linear regression is not suitable. Logistic regression is a widely used method for modelling categorical outcomes. This chapter introduces logistic regression, explains the assumptions it makes, and then illustrates how to perform logistic regression using practical examples. Finally, some common pitfalls are explained and methods for avoiding them are provided.

Intended learning outcomes

By the end of this chapter, you should be able to:

- understand why linear regression is not suitable for categorical outcomes;
- run a simple logistic regression model;
- interpret the results of logistic regression;
- add additional covariates to a model;
- perform likelihood ratio and Wald tests to compare two models;
- present results as probabilities.

Why linear regression is not suitable for dichotomous outcomes

When you have an outcome variable that is dichotomous, taking only two values, linear regression is not suitable. Examples of dichotomous variables are cardiovascular disease (yes/no), HIV status (positive, negative), hazardous alcohol drinking pattern (yes/no). Here is a hypothetical data set used to illustrate this point. It is data to study the possible association between financial hardship in midlife (the exposure) and common mental disorder in old age (the outcome), controlling for the possible confounding role of age.

Table 14.1 Example data for dichotomous variables

ID	Financial hardship	Age	Common mental disorder
1	0	35	0
2	1	55	1
3	1	57	1
4	1	63	0
5	0	45	0
6	1	65	1
7	0	52	1
8	1	66	1
9	0	40	0
10	0	68	0

You might think that linear regression can be used in exactly the same way, but it cannot. This can be illustrated in two ways. First, one of the key assumptions of linear regression is violated. Second, the interpretation of the beta coefficients is not valid.

Residuals are not normally distributed

```
data <- read.table('plate-dysphagia.csv', header=TRUE, sep=',')
attach(data)
head(data) #this shows the first few lines of data and the
# column headings
fit <- lm (dysphagia ~ age_years)
resid <- fit$residuals
sd.resid <- sd(resid)
stdres = rstandard(fit)
qqnorm(stdres, ylab="Standardised Residuals", xlab="Normal
Scores plotted against Standardized Residuals")
qqline(stdres)
```

You can see here that the residuals are not normally distributed, making the data unsuitable for linear regression.

One of the most important assumptions of linear regression is that the residuals are normally distributed. If they are not, then the beta estimates and standard errors are probably wrong.

The interpretation of the beta values is not valid

```
fit <- lm (dysphagia ~ plate+age_years+male)
summary(fit)
```

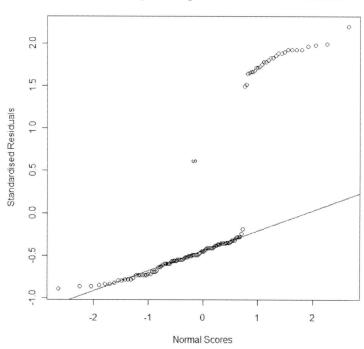

Figure 14.1 Plot showing that residuals are nor normally distributed for categorical outcomes using linear regression

Consider the model above, which is a linear regression of dysphagia, or difficulty swallowing (yes coded 1, no coded 0) on plate (described in Box 14.1), age and sex. The coefficient obtained is 0.2618 which is statistically significant, but what does the coefficient mean? It is the expected linear change in dysphagia per unit for those with a plate inserted compared to those without, holding age and sex constant. Yet we know that the outcome can only possibly be 0 or 1 – it cannot be 0.2618! The beta coefficient is not meaningful. We need to find a type of regression model that can handle categorical outcomes

Introducing logistic regression

Logistic regression is designed for modelling categorical outcomes with one or more predictor variables. It is ideally suited to the situation where you have an exposure, a set of confounders or possible mediators, and a categorical outcome. When running a logistic regression, you need to think about the probability that someone will experience the outcome, rather than their estimated value. We can for example, calculate the probability of having dysphagia or not having dysphagia. This produces a linear, graduated scale.

It is not meaningful to predict someone will have an outcome of dysphagia, but it is meaningful to say that they have a probability of 0.65 of experiencing the outcome, for example. Logistic regression will estimate the probability of the outcome, based on a non-linear function. It is therefore more suitable to categorical outcomes than linear regression.

The trouble with probabilities in this situation is that they can exceed 1 (e.g. 1.20). To address this, we transform the probability into an odds ratio. Odds ratios in logistic regression are interpreted in nearly exactly the same way as we have encountered before (e.g. in Chapter 4).

The trouble with odds ratios however, is that they cannot estimate scores below zero. To address this, we take the log. The log odds ratio is called the logit. The logit is not bounded at zero or one.

The trouble with logits, however, is that we cannot use ordinary least squares regression. To address this, we have to use software and maximum likelihood (ML) estimation to work out what the beta values are. ML is an iterative method, meaning that many different attempts are made to find the best values, which can take some time. For this and other reasons, ML is usually done using statistical software.

This may all sound very complicated, but since this is an introductory textbook, the most important thing to remember when starting out is that logistic (not linear) regression is needed when you have a dichotomous outcome and more than one predictor variable. Although logistic regression calculates probabilities of an outcome occurring, these are presented as logits and as odds ratios rather than probabilities. At the end of the chapter is a very brief explanation of how you can convert odds ratio to probabilities of an outcome occurring, following logistic regression.

Preparing for logistic regression

There are some important points you should remember about logistic regression:

- the model is intended to explain the effect of the predictor variables on the dichotomous outcome variable;

- the outcome is dichotomous or binary;

- predictor variables (exposure, covariates) can be either categorical or continuous;

- ff predictor variables are ordered categorical variables, you need to create dummy variables (see Chapter 13).

Logistic regression is not suitable for categorical outcomes that have more than two possible values. There are techniques available for such situations, including multinomial logistic regression, but these are beyond the scope of this book. Further reading around this topic is provided at the end of the chapter.

The logistic regression equation

The logistic regression equation looks very similar to the linear regression equation

$$\ln(\text{odds}) = \ln\left(\frac{\hat{p}}{1-\hat{p}}\right) = \beta_0 + x\beta_1$$

$\ln(\text{odds})$ is the log odds or 'logit'
x is the value of the predictor variable
β_0 is the intercept parameter
β_1 is the slope parameter
$\hat{p}$ is the probability of the outcome occurring (the 'hat' symbol indicates that this is the estimated probability, not the actual probability)

The key difference here is that the odds are calculated on a natural logarithmic scale. We calculate the log odds ratio (or 'logit'), not the odds ratio itself.

Recap: log odds, odds, probability

Table 14.2 Log odds, odds and probability

Log odds (logit)	Odds	p
−6.90676	0.001001	0.001
−0.59512	0.010101	0.01
−1.38629	0.25	0.2
−0.8473	0.428571	0.3
−0.40547	0.666667	0.4
0	1	0.5
0.405465	1.5	0.6
0.847298	2.333333	0.7
1.386294	4	0.8
2.197225	9	0.9
6.906755	999	0.999
9.21024	9999	0.9999

Box 14.1 Data set: surgical plate insertion during cervical spine surgery data and subsequent dysphagia

These data were used to evaluate whether inserting a plate during surgery would lead to dysphagia (difficulty swallowing). Cervical spine surgery can often lead to dysphagia. Some clinicians have wondered if the insertion of a surgical plate during surgery is a risk factor for subsequent dysphagia. The outcome (dependent) variable is a binary variable, which takes the value 0 if dysphagia was not reported following surgery, and 1 if dysphagia was reported. The exposure of interest is having a plate inserted, coded 0 if a plate was not inserted and 1 if a plate was inserted. We want to control (adjust) for age, sex, American Society of Anaesthesiologists (ASA) status score, having had previous neck surgery, and smoking status. The ASA score is a system for rating patients' suitability for surgery, developed by anaesthesiologists [106]:

1 normal and healthy;

2 mild systemic disease;

3 severe systemic disease;

4 severe life-threatening systemic disease;

5 moribund not expected to survive without operating;

6 brain-dead and organs to be removed for donor purposes.

A table of descriptive statistics is shown in Table 14.3, so that you can get a feel for the data. In the table, ASA status is treated as categorical. It shows the number and percentage of people classified as having severe/incapacitating systemic disease. In our logistic regression model however, we will treat ASA score as continuous. In reality however, it is an ordinal scale.

Data source: Dr. Jon Short

Getting started with logistic regression

Before we begin modelling, as always, it is sensible to create a table of descriptive statistics. In Table 14.3 we can see that dysphagia looks more likely among those patients who had a plate inserted, but this a descriptive result. We want to consider possible confounding factors (age, sex, ASA score, previous neck surgery, smoking).

The column percentages were used in this table, to show the proportion of people with the variable of interest in each group (no dysphagia, dysphagia). The chi-square test is used to test the independence of categorical predictor variables (i.e. the exposure and covariates, listed in the first column) and the categorical outcome variable (dysphagia).

Box 14.2 R code: comparing categorial study variables according to dysphagia status

```
mytable<-table(plate, dysphagia)
mytable
prop.table(mytable, 2) #2 indicates column percentages
# (change to 1 for row percentages)
chisq.test(mytable)
```

Table 14.3 Descriptive statistics for study variables according to dysphagia status

	No dysphagia (n = 94) n (%)	Dysphagia (n = 28) n (%)	Total (n = 122) n (%)	p a
Plate	19 (20.1)	15 (53.6)	34 (27.9)	0.001
Male	57 (60.6)	14 (50.0)	71 (58.2)	0.43
ASA status = severe or incapacitating	23 (24.5)	9 (32.1)	32 (26.2)	0.57
Previous neck surgery	13 (13.8)	7 (25.0)	20 (16.4)	0.27
Current regular smoker	37 (39.4)	9 (32.1)	46 (37.7)	0.64
	Mean (SD)	Mean (SD)	Mean (SD)	b
Age (range 27 to 84)	53.24 (12.7)	58.21 (11.82)	54.39 (12.63)	0.07

a = Chi-square test for differences in proportions, b = *t*-test for differences in means.

The code in Box 14.2 was repeated for each variable (male, ASA status, previous neck surgery etc.)

For the continuous variable age_years, the mean and standard deviation were obtained separately for each group using the subset option, which runs the command requests only on a subset of the data (here, those without dysphagia and then those with dysphagia separately) (Box 14.3)

Box 14.3 R code: comparing continuous study variables according to dysphagia status

```
mean(subset(data$age_years, dysphagia ==0))
mean(subset(data$age_years, dysphagia ==1))
sd(subset(data$age_years, dysphagia ==0))
sd(subset(data$age_years, dysphagia ==1))
```

Results from a simple logistic regression model

This model contains plate, age and sex. It is a 'minimally adjusted' model, because we consider that age and sex are key confounding factors.

Box 14.4 R code for logistic regression

```
library(aod) #remember that if a package such as aod is not
# installed, you need to install it first
library(ggplot2)
data <- read.table('plate-dysphagia.csv', header=TRUE,
sep=',')
attach(data)
#basic model (minimally adjusted for age and sex)
mylogit <- glm(dysphagia ~ plate + age_years + male , data =
data, family = "binomial")
```

```
Call:
glm(formula = dysphagia_c ~ plate_c + age_years + male, family = "binomial",
    data = data)

Deviance Residuals:
    Min        1Q    Median        3Q       Max
-1.3083   -0.6256   -0.5407   -0.4496    2.2059

Coefficients:
              Estimate Std. Error z value Pr(>|z|)
(Intercept)   -2.31321    1.09482  -2.113   0.0346 *
plate_c        1.33069    0.51162   2.601   0.0093 **
age_years      0.01669    0.02117   0.788   0.4306
male          -0.54530    0.48238  -1.130   0.2583
---
Signif. codes:  0 '***' 0.001 '**' 0.01 '*' 0.05 '.' 0.1 ' ' 1

(Dispersion parameter for binomial family taken to be 1)

    Null deviance: 131.44  on 121  degrees of freedom
Residual deviance: 118.85  on 118  degrees of freedom
AIC: 126.85

Number of Fisher Scoring iterations: 4
```

Figure 14.2 R output for logistic regression

The 'Call' shown at the start of the output in Figure 14.2 is simply a reminder of what model we asked for. You can see that R has repeated the syntax we specified for this model.

The deviance residuals are a measure of goodness-of-fit for the model. This is not particularly useful except when you want to compare the goodness-of-fit of competing models, described below.

The coefficients are shown next, and are the most important part of the output. The estimates, their standard errors, a z-statistic (Wald statistic) and a p-value are shown in columns. In rows, we have the intercept, the exposure (whether a plate was inserted), and two covariates (age and male).

The intercept is the log odds for those without a plate inserted, who are age 0 and are female.

Note that the coefficients refer to expected changes in the log odds (logits) of an outcome occurring, they are not odds ratios.

Information on how to create model-estimated probabilities is given at the end of this chapter.

Next, we will break down the modelling process in order to better understand what is happening. First, we will explore a simple logistic regression model that has no predictor variables. Then we will run a model containing only the exposure. Finally, we will add our proposed confounding factors.

Logistic regression: intercept only

In order to understand the intercept in logistic regression, it may help to think about a basic logistic regression that contains no predictors. This code will produce such a model, but note that R will automatically drop dysphagia as a predictor variable, knowing that this is not possible. Dysphagia is only

```
> mytable<-table(dysphagia)
> mytable
dysphagia
 0  1
94 28
> prop.table(mytable) #gives cell proportions
dysphagia
          0         1
0.7704918 0.2295082
>
> |
```

Figure 14.3 R output showing proportion of patients with dysphagia

mentioned because we have to name at least one predictor variable in order to get the model to run. You can therefore ignore the warning message that 'the response appeared on the right-hand side and was dropped'.

```
intercept <- glm(dysphagia ~ dysphagia, data = data, family =
"binomial")
summary(intercept)
```

This produces an intercept value of –1.2111. Because $\log(p/(1–p)) = -1.2111$, p is the overall probability of having dysphagia. This will correspond to a simple frequency table of the dysphagia variable.

```
mytable<-table(dysphagia)
mytable
prop.table(mytable) #gives cell proportions
```

$$\log(0.2295/(1–0.2295)) = -1.2111$$

The intercept is the log odds of having dysphagia for the entire study population. The odds of having dysphagia is $\exp(-1.2111) = 0.2979$. The probability of having dysphagia is $0.2979/(1 + 0.2979) = 0.2295$ or 23 per cent.

Logistic regression: exposure only

In this model, we will use the exposure (plate) without any adjustment for covariates. This is purely to illustrate how a basic model works. In reality, we would nearly always want to adjust for a minimal set of covariates such as age and sex. It is always sensible to cross-tabulate your exposure and outcome variable beforehand, to check that the data look suitable for logistic regression. As above:

```
mytable<-table(plate, dysphagia)
mytable
prop.table(mytable, 2) #2 indicates column percentages (change
# to 1 for row percentages)
```

This shows that there are no empty cells, which would cause problems in trying to run the model. If you want, use the standard method for calculating the odds of dysphagia in each group (plate, no plate), but remember that we have not adjusted for any confounding factors yet.

	Dysphagia	No dysphagia
Plate	15	19
No plate	13	75

- for patients who had a plate inserted, the odds are: (15/19) = 0.7895;

- for patients who had no plate inserted, the odds are: (13/75) 0.1733;

- the odds ratio for dysphagia is therefore: 0.7895/0.1733 = 4.56.

Now compare this to the output obtained from logistic regression.

```
intercept <- glm(dysphagia ~ plate, data = data, family =
"binomial")
summary(intercept)
```

The intercept is –1.7525 and this is the log odds for those without a plate inserted, because they are the reference group.

We previously calculated the odds for those without a plate to be 0.1733. The log odds is log(0.1733) = –1.7525 which corresponds to the output obtained from R.

```
>
> intercept <- glm(dysphagia ~ plate, data = data, family = "binomial")
> summary(intercept)

Call:
glm(formula = dysphagia ~ plate, family = "binomial", data = data)

Deviance Residuals:
    Min      1Q  Median      3Q     Max
-1.0788  -0.5654  -0.5654  -0.5654  1.9557

Coefficients:
            Estimate Std. Error z value Pr(>|z|)
(Intercept)  -1.7525     0.3004  -5.833 5.43e-09 ***
plate         1.5161     0.4578   3.312 0.000926 ***
---
Signif. codes:  0 '***' 0.001 '**' 0.01 '*' 0.05 '.' 0.1 ' ' 1

(Dispersion parameter for binomial family taken to be 1)

    Null deviance: 131.44  on 121  degrees of freedom
Residual deviance: 120.36  on 120  degrees of freedom
AIC: 124.36

Number of Fisher Scoring iterations: 4
```

Figure 14.4 R output for logistic regression: exposure only

269

The coefficient for 'plate' is the log of the odds ratio comparing the group who received a plate with those who did not: 1.5161. To obtain the odds ratio, simply take the exponent of this log odds ratio: exp(1.5161) = 4.56.

Logistic regression: exposure and covariates

When adding covariate (e.g. age and sex). The coefficients obtained in the output are adjusted (controlled, held constant) for other predictors in the model. So the coefficient for plate in our next model is the log odds ratio for plate, holding age and sex constant. Similarly, the coefficients for age and sex are the expected change in the log odds (logit), holding other variables in the model constant. We often call this model the 'minimally adjusted' model because it necessary to control for age and sex in many situations.

```
#basic model (minimally adjusted for age and sex)
mylogit <- glm(dysphagia ~ plate + age_years + male , data =
data, family = "binomial")
summary(mylogit)
```

- The coefficient of 1.33 for plate corresponds to an odds ratio of 3.78 (95% CI 1.39, 10.31), adjusting for age and sex. This could be considered the minimally adjusted odds ratio. It is consistent with an increase in the odds of dysphagia for patients who had a plate inserted.

```
> summary(mylogit)

Call:
glm(formula = dysphagia ~ plate + age_years + male, family = "binomial",
    data = data)

Deviance Residuals:
    Min       1Q   Median       3Q      Max
-1.3083  -0.6256  -0.5407  -0.4496   2.2059

Coefficients:
            Estimate Std. Error z value Pr(>|z|)
(Intercept) -2.31321    1.09482  -2.113   0.0346 *
plate        1.33069    0.51162   2.601   0.0093 **
age_years    0.01669    0.02117   0.788   0.4306
male        -0.54530    0.48238  -1.130   0.2583
---
Signif. codes:  0 '***' 0.001 '**' 0.01 '*' 0.05 '.' 0.1 ' ' 1

(Dispersion parameter for binomial family taken to be 1)

    Null deviance: 131.44  on 121  degrees of freedom
Residual deviance: 118.85  on 118  degrees of freedom
AIC: 126.85

Number of Fisher Scoring iterations: 4

> |
```

Figure 14.5 R output for logisitic regression: exposure and covariates

- The coefficient for age_years of 0.01669 refers to the expected increase in the log odds of dysphagia per increase in year of age. It is not statistically significant.

- The coefficient for male f -0.5453 is the expected change in the log odds of dysphagia comparing males to females. It is consistent with lower odds of dysphagia for males, but is not statistically significant.

Next, we will consider other possible confounding factors and add these to the model.

Comparing the goodness of fit of two logistic regression models: loglikelihood test

Suppose we want to compare the fit of our minimally adjusted model (plate, age, sex) and a more complex model, than contains further covariates. We can compare the fit by conducting a likelihood ratio test. This subtracts the loglikelihood value of the nested model from that of the comparison model, and multiplies the difference by two. The resulting scores from this equation happen to have a chi-square distribution. This means that we can find out if a model is significantly different from another, using a chi-square table to test the null hypothesis. There is 1 degree of freedom in most cases, because we tend to test the fit of a model that has one additional predictor variable.

- $L_{RT} = 2(L_1 - L_0)$;
- L_1 = contains the variable you are interested in;
- L_0 = contains the model without the variable .

In practice, this test is performed by statistical software in most situations.

```
library(lmtest)
model1 <- glm(dysphagia ~ plate + age_years + male, data =
data, family = "binomial")
summary(model1)
model2 <- glm(dysphagia ~ plate + age_years + male + asa, data
= data, family = "binomial")
summary(model2)
lrtest(model2,model1) #the first model is said to be nested
# within the second
```

Model 2 does not fit the data significantly better than Model 1, so it may be unnecessary to add ASA score to the model.

We might want to consider adding smoking and previous neck surgery to the model.

```
> lrtest(model2,model1) #the first model is said to be nested within the second
Likelihood ratio test

Model 1: dysphagia ~ plate + age_years + male + asa
Model 2: dysphagia ~ plate + age_years + male
  #Df  LogLik Df  Chisq Pr(>Chisq)
1   5 -59.059
2   4 -59.424 -1 0.7293     0.3931
>
```

Figure 14.6 R code for likelihood ratio test, comparing models 1 and 2

```
> lrtest(model3,model1) #compares model3 and model1
Likelihood ratio test

Model 1: dysphagia ~ plate + age_years + male + smoker + prevneck
Model 2: dysphagia ~ plate + age_years + male
  #Df  LogLik Df  Chisq Pr(>Chisq)
1   6 -59.287
2   4 -59.424 -2 0.2743     0.8719
> |
```

Figure 14.7 R code for likelihood ratio test, comparing models 1 and 3

```
model3 <- glm(dysphagia ~ plate + age_years + male + smoker
+ prevneck, data = data, family = "binomial")
summary(model3)
lrtest(model3,model1) #compares model3 and model1
```

Model 3 does not fit significantly better than Model 1, so we may conclude that Model 1 is a sufficiently parsimonious model of the data. Plate insertion during surgery is associated with dysphagia, independently of age, sex, ASA score, smoking and previous neck surgery. Note however, that you should avoid evaluating the fit of models by repeatedly re-running them after adding different variables. This can be interpreted as 'pre-screening' your data to see which variables are significant. A related technique called stepwise regression has also received similar criticism [84]. It is arguably better, in most situations, to decide beforehand which variables should be in your model and why. Then run the analysis as planned, and do not re-run analysis unless there is good reason to do so. For example, you might want to compare the fit of a model containing smoking and one without, in order to determine if smoking is an informative variable for prediction purposes. You should report that you have done this comparison however, so that your results describe what actually happened.

Identifying whether a variable significantly improves fit of the model: Wald test

The Wald test is useful if you want to compare whether two regression coefficients are zero. If the Wald test fails to reject this assumption, the variables appear not to be particularly useful because they are unnecessary in the model.

```
> wald.test(b = coef(mylogit), Sigm
Wald test:
----------

Chi-squared test:
X2 = 2.3, df = 3, P(> X2) = 0.51
>
```

Figure 14.8 Wald test: logistic regression

```
#this example is adapted from the UCLA web page: http://www.
# ats.ucla.edu/stat/r/dae/logit.htm
data <- read.table('plate-dysphagia.csv', header=TRUE, sep=',')
attach(data)
head(data)
library(aod)
library(ggplot2)
xtabs(~dysphagia + plate, data = data)
data$asa <- factor(data$asa)
mylogit <- glm(dysphagia ~ plate + age_years + male + asa, data
= data, family = "binomial")
summary(mylogit)
confint.default(mylogit) #obtain confidence intervals
exp(cbind(OR = coef(mylogit), confint(mylogit))) #odds ratios
wald.test(b = coef(mylogit), Sigma = vcov(mylogit), Terms =
3:5) #This tests whether the 3rd-5th coefficients in the model
# significantly improve the fit of the model
```

The effect of ASA score is shown to be not statistically significant.

Obtaining predicted probabilities

```
data$plate <- factor(data$plate)
mylogit <- glm(dysphagia ~ plate + age_years + male, data
= data, family = "binomial")
summary(mylogit)
newdata1 <- with(data, data.frame( age_years = mean(age_
years), male = 1, plate = factor(0:1)))
newdata1$rankP <- predict(mylogit, newdata = newdata1,
type = "response")
newdata1
```

This shows the estimated probability of having subsequent dysphagia for those with and without a plate insertion, at mean age (54.39 years) and for men. It is necessary to specify some value for covariates in the model, so that the probability is conditional on all variables included in the original model. Many people find these probabilities easier to understand than odds ratios. If you publish your research, reviewers might find the following statement more readily interpretable than odds ratios:

```
> newdata1 <- with(data, data.frame( age_years = mean(age_years), male = 1, plate = factor(0:1)))
> newdata1$rankP <- predict(mylogit, newdata = newdata1, type = "response")
> newdata1
  age_years male plate      rankP
1  54.38525    1     0 0.1244573
2  54.38525    1     1 0.3497378
>
```

Figure 14.9 Predicted probabilities following logistic regression

For men at age 55, the probability of dysphagia was 12.5% if they had no plate inserted during surgery, but it was 35.0% if they did have a plate inserted.

Note however, that you must report odds ratios and confidence intervals as your main results – readers will expect to see these.

Summary

In this chapter you have been introduced to logistic regression, a technique widely used in the health sciences to predict categorical outcomes from a set of predictors. The predictors can be continuous, categorical or a mixture. One of them is usually the exposure of interest, the others are considered covariates. Covariates can be confounding variables or possible mediators. The choice of covariates should be guided by prior research, theory and existing knowledge.

Further reading

Tabachnick B, Fidell L: *Using Multivariate Statistics*: Pearson Education; 2007.
Hosmer D, Lemeshow S: *Applied logistic regression*: Wiley Interscience; 2000.

Critical values for the *t*-test

df	One-tailed significance 0.05	0.025	0.01	0.005
	Two-tailed significance 0.1	0.05	0.02	0.01
2	2.920	4.303	6.965	9.925
3	2.353	3.182	4.541	5.841
4	2.132	2.776	3.747	4.604
5	2.015	2.571	3.365	4.032
6	1.943	2.447	3.365	3.708
7	1.895	2.365	2.998	3.500
8	1.860	2.306	2.897	3.355
9	1.833	2.262	2.821	3.250
10	1.813	2.228	2.764	3.169
11	1.796	2.201	2.718	3.106
12	1.782	2.179	2.681	3.055
13	1.771	2.160	2.650	3.012
14	1.761	2.145	2.625	2.977
15	1.753	2.132	2.603	2.947
16	1.746	2.120	2.583	2.921
17	1.740	2.110	2.567	2.898
18	1.734	2.101	2.552	2.878
19	1.729	2.093	2.539	2.861
20	1.725	2.086	2.528	2.845
21	1.721	2.080	2.518	2.831
22	1.717	2.074	2.508	2.819
23	1.714	2.069	2.500	2.807
24	1.711	2.064	2.492	2.797
25	1.708	2.064	2.485	2.787
26	1.706	2.055	2.479	2.779
27	1.703	2.052	2.473	2.771
28	1.701	2.048	2.467	2.763
29	1.699	2.045	2.462	2.756
30	1.697	2.042	2.457	2.750
35	1.690	2.030	2.438	2.724
40	1.684	2.021	2.423	2.704
45	1.679	2.014	2.412	2.690
50	1.676	2.009	2.403	2.678
55	1.673	2.004	2.396	2.668
60	1.671	2.000	2.090	2.660
65	1.669	1.997	2.385	2.654
70	1.667	1.994	2.381	2.648
75	1.665	1.992	2.377	2.643
80	1.664	1.990	2.374	2.639
85	1.663	1.988	2.371	2.635
90	1.662	1.987	2.369	2.632
95	1.661	1.985	2.366	2.629
100	1.660	1.984	2.364	2.626
200	1.653	1.972	2.345	2.601
300	1.650	1.968	2.339	2.592
400	1.649	1.966	2.336	2.588
500	1.648	1.965	2.334	2.586
1000	1.646	1.962	2.330	2.581
∞	1.645	1.960	2.326	2.576

Appendix 2
Critical values for the *F*-test

F distribution critical values for $p = 0.05$

	1	2	3	4	5	6	7	8	9	10
3	10.128	9.552	9.277	9.117	9.013	8.941	8.887	8.845	8.812	8.785
4	7.709	6.944	6.591	6.388	6.256	6.163	6.094	6.041	5.999	5.964
5	6.608	5.786	5.409	5.192	5.050	4.950	4.876	4.818	4.772	4.735
6	5.987	5.143	4.757	4.534	4.387	4.284	4.207	4.147	4.099	4.060
7	5.591	4.737	4.347	4.120	3.972	3.866	3.787	3.726	3.677	3.637
8	5.318	4.459	4.066	3.838	3.688	3.581	3.500	3.438	3.388	3.347
9	5.117	4.256	3.863	3.633	3.482	3.374	3.293	3.230	3.179	3.137
10	4.965	4.103	3.708	3.478	3.326	3.217	3.135	3.072	3.020	2.978
15	4.543	3.682	3.287	3.056	2.901	2.790	2.707	2.641	2.588	2.544
20	4.351	3.493	3.098	2.866	2.711	2.599	2.514	2.447	2.393	2.348
25	4.242	3.385	2.991	2.759	2.603	2.490	2.405	2.337	2.282	2.236
30	4.171	3.316	2.922	2.690	2.534	2.421	2.334	2.266	2.211	2.165
35	4.121	3.267	2.874	2.641	2.485	2.372	2.285	2.217	2.161	2.114
40	4.085	3.232	2.839	2.606	2.449	2.336	2.249	2.180	2.124	2.077
45	4.057	3.204	2.812	2.579	2.422	2.308	2.221	2.152	2.096	2.049
50	4.034	3.183	2.790	2.557	2.400	2.286	2.199	2.130	2.073	2.026
60	4.001	3.150	2.758	2.525	2.368	2.254	2.167	2.097	2.040	1.993
70	3.978	3.128	2.736	2.503	2.346	2.231	2.143	2.074	2.017	1.969
80	3.960	3.111	2.719	2.486	2.329	2.214	2.126	2.056	1.999	1.951
90	3.947	3.098	2.706	2.473	2.316	2.201	2.113	2.043	1.986	1.938
100	3.936	3.087	2.696	2.463	2.305	2.191	2.103	2.032	1.975	1.927

Appendix 3
Table of z-values

Critical values of the normal distribution (source: [115])

z	0.00	0.01	0.02	0.03	0.04	0.05	0.06	0.07	0.08	0.09
0.0	0.0000	0.0040	0.0080	0.0120	0.0160	0.0199	0.0239	0.0279	0.0319	0.0359
0.1	0.0398	0.0438	0.0478	0.0517	0.0557	0.0596	0.0636	0.0675	0.0714	0.0753
0.2	0.0793	0.0832	0.0871	0.0910	0.0948	0.0987	0.1026	0.1064	0.1103	0.1141
0.3	0.1179	0.1217	0.1255	0.1293	0.1331	0.1368	0.1406	0.1443	0.1480	0.1517
0.4	0.1554	0.1591	0.1628	0.1664	0.1700	0.1736	0.1772	0.1808	0.1844	0.1879
0.5	0.1915	0.1950	0.1985	0.2019	0.2054	0.2088	0.2123	0.2157	0.2190	0.2224
0.6	0.2257	0.2291	0.2324	0.2357	0.2389	0.2422	0.2454	0.2486	0.2517	0.2549
0.7	0.2580	0.2611	0.2642	0.2673	0.2704	0.2734	0.2764	0.2794	0.2823	0.2852
0.8	0.2881	0.2910	0.2939	0.2967	0.2995	0.3023	0.3051	0.3078	0.3106	0.3133
0.9	0.3159	0.3186	0.3212	0.3238	0.3264	0.3289	0.3315	0.3340	0.3365	0.3389
1.0	0.3413	0.3438	0.3461	0.3485	0.3508	0.3531	0.3554	0.3577	0.3599	0.3621
1.1	0.3643	0.3665	0.3686	0.3708	0.3729	0.3749	0.3770	0.3790	0.3810	0.3830
1.2	0.3849	0.3869	0.3888	0.3907	0.3925	0.3944	0.3962	0.3980	0.3997	0.4015
1.3	0.4032	0.4049	0.4066	0.4082	0.4099	0.4115	0.4131	0.4147	0.4162	0.4177
1.4	0.4192	0.4207	0.4222	0.4236	0.4251	0.4265	0.4279	0.4292	0.4306	0.4319
1.5	0.4332	0.4345	0.4357	0.4370	0.4382	0.4394	0.4406	0.4418	0.4429	0.4441
1.6	0.4452	0.4463	0.4474	0.4484	0.4495	0.4505	0.4515	0.4525	0.4535	0.4545
1.7	0.4554	0.4564	0.4573	0.4582	0.4591	0.4599	0.4608	0.4616	0.4625	0.4633
1.8	0.4641	0.4649	0.4656	0.4664	0.4671	0.4678	0.4686	0.4693	0.4699	0.4706
1.9	0.4713	0.4719	0.4726	0.4732	0.4738	0.4744	0.4750	0.4756	0.4761	0.4767
2.0	0.4772	0.4778	0.4783	0.4788	0.4793	0.4798	0.4803	0.4808	0.4812	0.4817
2.1	0.4821	0.4826	0.4830	0.4834	0.4838	0.4842	0.4846	0.4850	0.4854	0.4857
2.2	0.4861	0.4864	0.4868	0.4871	0.4875	0.4878	0.4881	0.4884	0.4887	0.4890
2.3	0.4893	0.4896	0.4898	0.4901	0.4904	0.4906	0.4909	0.4911	0.4913	0.4916
2.4	0.4918	0.4920	0.4922	0.4925	0.4927	0.4929	0.4931	0.4932	0.4934	0.4936
2.5	0.4938	0.4940	0.4941	0.4943	0.4945	0.4946	0.4948	0.4949	0.4951	0.4952
2.6	0.4953	0.4955	0.4956	0.4957	0.4959	0.4960	0.4961	0.4962	0.4963	0.4964
2.7	0.4965	0.4966	0.4967	0.4968	0.4969	0.4970	0.4971	0.4972	0.4973	0.4974
2.8	0.4974	0.4975	0.4976	0.4977	0.4977	0.4978	0.4979	0.4979	0.4980	0.4981
2.9	0.4981	0.4982	0.4982	0.4983	0.4984	0.4984	0.4985	0.4985	0.4986	0.4986
3.0	0.4987	0.4987	0.4987	0.4988	0.4988	0.4989	0.4989	0.4989	0.4990	0.4990

Appendix 4
T/U table for Mann Whitney U test

N_B	1	2	3	4	5	6	7	8	9	10	11	12	13	14	15	16	17	18	19	20
N_A																				
1	–	–	–	–	–	–	–	–	–	–	–	–	–	–	–	–	–	–	–	–
2	–	–	–	–	–	–	–	0	0	0	0	1	1	1	1	1	2	2	2	2
3	–	–	–	–	0	1	1	2	2	3	3	4	4	5	5	6	6	7	7	8
4	–	–	–	0	1	2	3	4	4	5	6	7	8	9	10	11	11	12	13	13
5	–	–	0	1	2	3	5	6	7	8	9	10	12	13	14	15	17	18	19	20
6	–	–	–	–	–	5	6	8	10	11	13	14	16	17	19	21	22	24	25	27
7	–	–	–	–	–	–	8	10	12	14	16	18	20	22	24	26	28	30	32	34
8	–	–	–	–	–	–	–	13	15	17	19	22	24	26	29	31	34	36	38	41
9	–	–	–	–	–	–	–	–	17	20	23	26	28	31	34	37	39	42	45	48
10	–	–	–	–	–	–	–	–	–	23	26	29	33	36	39	42	45	48	52	55
11	–	–	–	–	–	–	–	–	–	–	30	33	37	40	44	47	51	55	58	62
12	–	–	–	–	–	–	–	–	–	–	–	37	41	45	49	53	57	61	65	69
13	–	–	–	–	–	–	–	–	–	–	–	–	45	50	54	59	63	67	72	76
14	–	–	–	–	–	–	–	–	–	–	–	–	–	55	59	64	67	74	78	83
15	–	–	–	–	–	–	–	–	–	–	–	–	–	–	64	70	75	80	85	90
16	–	–	–	–	–	–	–	–	–	–	–	–	–	–	–	75	81	86	92	98
17	–	–	–	–	–	–	–	–	–	–	–	–	–	–	–	–	87	93	99	105
18	–	–	–	–	–	–	–	–	–	–	–	–	–	–	–	–	–	99	106	112
19	–	–	–	–	–	–	–	–	–	–	–	–	–	–	–	–	–	–	113	119
20	–	–	–	–	–	–	–	–	–	–	–	–	–	–	–	–	–	–	–	127

Appendix 5
Critical values for the Wilcoxon test

N	One-tailed test 0.025 / Two-tailed test 0.05	0.01 / 0.02	0.05 / 0.01
6	2	1	
7	4	2	
8	6	4	0
9	8	4	2
10	11	8	3
11	14	11	5
12	17	14	7
13	21	17	10
14	26	21	13
15	31	25	16
16	36	30	20
17	42	35	24
18	47	40	28
19	54	46	33
20	60	52	37
21	68	59	42
22	76	66	47
23	84	74	54
24	92	81	60
25	101	90	67

Appendix 6
Consent form

Anonymous Identification Number for this study:

CONSENT FORM

Title of Project:

Name of Researcher:

Initial box

1 I confirm that I have read and understand the above participant information sheet and have had the opportunity to ask questions.

2 I understand that my participation is voluntary and that I am free to withdraw at any time without giving any reason without my legal rights being affected.

3   I agree to take part in the above study.

_____

Print your name

_____

Signature and date

Appendix 7
Statistical power

A statistical power calculation tells us that for a given effect size, and a given sample size, the probability of avoiding a type II error (a 'false negative' result). Traditionally researchers try to have power at 80 per cent, so that there is a 20 per cent chance of missing an effect that is actually there in reality.

- Effect size. The size of the effect we want to detect. Some researchers have arbitrarily defined these as 'small', 'medium' and 'large' but this is not recommended. Instead, we should think about the clinical and public health significance of the effect. If a reduction of half a standard deviation in a measure of psychological distress, for example, is considered important for the population, then this is the effect size we should be concerned with. Interventions may have small effects, which can have considerable benefit when applied at the population level. Research studies should have the power to detect such effects, or they may be missed.

- Type I error. The null hypothesis (no effect) is true, but researchers conclude that there is an effect. This usually happens because the alpha value is set at .05, corresponding to the traditional p-value of .05. This means that 5 per cent of the time, p-values <.05 are found by chance.

- Type II error. The null hypothesis is false (there is an effect), but researchers conclude that there is no effect. This usually happens because the sample size is not large enough to detect the effect.

- Alpha. The probability of incorrectly rejecting the null hypothesis, .05 or 5 per cent. Sometimes called a "false positive" result, or a result that is due to chance.

- Beta. The probability of incorrectly retaining the null hypothesis. This is arguably more serious, because there was an effect but we didn't find one. A statistical power calculation reduces the risk of making this kind of error.

- Statistical power. Statistical power is $1 - \beta$, or "1 minus the probability of making a type II error", which is .80 or 80 per cent.

		Reality	
		H_0 True	H_0 False
Research findings	H_0 True	☺	☹ Type II Error $\beta = 0.20$
	H_0 False	☹ Type I Error $\alpha = 0.05$	☺

Appendix 8
Validity and bias

Validity

There are two kinds of validity, external and internal [108]:

- Internal validity is defined as the extent to which systematic error (bias) is not present during data collection. Bias is when error produces results that are consistently pushed in one direction because of non-random variables.

- External validity is defined as the extent to which results generalise to other participants, settings, follow-up times and so on.

Taken together, both kinds of validity allow researchers to be confident that the claims they are making about their findings are justified. It is possible for a study to have good internal validity, and yet not generalise to a wider population (this is discussed in more detail in Chapter 9 on cohort studies). It may still have perfectly useful results. However, if a study has poor internal validity, external validity becomes irrelevant – an internally invalid study cannot generalise because bias is present:

> External validity is the degree to which the conclusions in a study would hold for other persons in other places and at other times. As such, internal validity is a prerequisite for external validity. [109]

We can therefore say that internal validity is necessary, but not sufficient, for external validity. There are several kinds of internal validity which are now discussed.

Confounding bias

Confounding is an important source of internal bias. It is important to eliminate confounding as far as possible. Possible strategies include: randomisation of the exposure across groups (e.g. randomised controlled trials), stratification into different levels of the confounder (e.g. cohort/observational studies), adjustment for the confounder using regression methods (Chapter 13). Confounding is a greater cause for concern in observational and cross-sectional studies than in RCTs. Addressing confounding is an important prerequisite for establishing causality (exposure x caused y, and this is not due to confounding factor a), and the ability to make causal inferences implies high internal validity.

Selection bias

Selection bias occurs when participants are put into groups for a study, and this is not done randomly. For example, suppose a doctor is investigating whether a new treatment x improves survival time for cancer patients. She might select patients with the worst prognosis to get the new treatment. This is perfectly understandable from a clinical viewpoint, but it would introduce selection bias. If the treatment group is compared to a control group who do not receive the new treatment, the groups need to be created randomly. Randomised controlled trials are designed for exactly this reason (Chapter 8). It is also important, if the group to which patients belong has changed, that data are analysed in the way originally intended. That is, the data should be analysed according to treatment intention. This method is called intention to treat (ITT) analysis. There are several types of selection bias [110]:

Nonresponse bias

Participants may be eligible for a study but may never respond to an invitation to participate. This introduces selection bias because we never get information about these people. As an example, lower socioeconomic groups are more likely to be non-responders. This means we have less information about them. Some researchers 'over-sample' low SES groups in order to address this problem.

Hospital admission bias

Participants with diseases who are in hospital are more likely to have co-morbidities (other illnesses) and are more likely to have unhealthy behaviours. This introduces selection bias, as is particularly problematic in case-control studies (Chapter 10). In case-control studies, the following situation is an example of Berkson's paradox [111], a form of hospital admission bias:

- the association will be distortedly larger if controls are from community-dwelling settings rather than hospital settings;

- the association will be distortedly smaller if controls do not have the disease but are from hospital settings.

The solution is to select both cases and controls from community settings, rather than hospital settings. However, this is often unrealistic and impractical [111].

Exclusion bias

Researchers may exclude certain groups in order to address confounding. For example, we might want to investigate the association between caffeine consumption and cardiovascular disease risk, and decide to exclude people with prevalent (existing) CVD at the baseline of the study. This would remove confounding by prevalent CVD but would introduce exclusion bias, because information about these people is not included in the analysis.

Awareness/publicity bias

Awareness bias occurs when participants are aware of a possible or claimed association between an exposure and disease, perhaps because media reports have raised their concern. Members of the public may be more likely to report exposure to industry, heavy mobile phone usage, pollutants and so on, if the media has raised their awareness of possible harmful effects. One example illustrating the possible impact of awareness bias comes from a study that found concern about illness was a stronger predictor of self-reported illness than was actual proximity to emissions from industrial outlets [112]. Awareness bias can be addressed by objective measures of exposure and outcome. In summary, left unchecked, selection bias can distort an association between exposure x and outcome y, because of how participants were selected.

Attrition bias and loss to follow-up

Attrition bias can result from loss to follow-up, although loss to follow-up itself does not imply bias. Loss to follow-up is when participants drop out of a study (attrition) [108]. This can occur because the participant has decided to drop out, because they are uncountable, or because the study team have decided not to contact them for some other reason. In a trial comparing, for example, a new treatment x with an existing treatment, we would want to follow patients up to see what their health outcomes were. It is perfectly normal for people to drop out. The question is, are those patients who have dropped out different from those who remained in the study? If they are different, then attrition bias could be present. For example, if we were investigating the success of a new treatment designed to stop people from smoking, and the heaviest, most committed smokers dropped out (perhaps they were less interested in quitting), we might falsely conclude that the treatment appeared to be more successful than it really was. The smokers who were verified as quitters happened to be the ones who were more interested in quitting, and so they remained in the study. Two kinds of attrition bias are particularly common:

Healthy survivor bias

Healthy participants tend to stay in a longitudinal study, which can distort the association between x and y. For example, healthy participants who smoke could introduce apparent 'healthy smoker effects', incorrectly suggesting that smoking is less hazardous for health outcomes than it really is (because the more unhealthy smokers have dropped out). This situation is sometimes called 'health selection', implying that participants have been unintentionally 'selected' for having healthier characteristics.

Healthy volunteer bias

Participants who are healthy may have higher levels of interest in health, health consciousness, health literacy and health knowledge. For these reasons, they may be more likely to participate and then remain in health research than people who are less healthy. This introduces healthy volunteer effects, worrying for cross-sectional studies (if healthier people agreed to take part) and additionally for longitudinal studies with repeated follow-ups (if healthier people agreed to continue taking part).

In trials, attrition bias can be addressed by imputing missing data (e.g. one method involves using the last known value of the health outcome) which is sometimes combined with ITT. In cohort studies (Chapter 9), attrition bias can be evaluated by comparing the characteristics of people who remained in the study to characteristics at recruitment, by imputing missing data, or by techniques that 'weight' the data to take drop out into account. These techniques are controversial but are often better than ignoring missing data or drawing conclusions based only on people with complete data.

Performance and detection bias

Performance bias occurs in a trial if participants who receive a new treatment are also given additional treatments. A similar kind of bias can occur if outcomes are more likely to be monitored by staff who know which treatment group patients are in, called detection bias. Both kinds of bias can easily be prevented by blinding patients and staff involved in a trial [108], so that no one knows which participants are receiving the new drug. Not all treatments can be blinded however, as we saw in Chapter 8. When blinding is not present, additional treatments could happen unintentionally. For example, if a nurse knows that a patient is receiving a new drug x for treating depression, he might spend slightly longer talking to the patient about his situation, and keep a closer eye on monitoring the patient over time. Has the drug or the additional support from the nurse influenced the improvement in the patient's mental health? Bias has been introduced into the study.

Observer bias

Observer bias can occur when members of the research team know the exposure status of a participant, and are involved in classifying the outcome. For example, a participant known to have a history of heavy alcohol drinking might be more likely to receive a diagnosis of alcoholic cirrhosis of the liver if the pathologist knows about their drinking habits [113].

Information bias

Information bias concerns measurement error. Has the exposure been measured correctly? Has the outcome been measured correctly? Think back to the 2 × 2 tables used to introduce odds ratios in Chapter 4. Suppose that the exposure x was smoking and the outcome y was lung cancer. If a number of smokers were misclassified as non-smokers (e.g. because they smoked but self-reported that they were a non-smoker), then they would be in the wrong cell of the table. Similarly, if the outcome was not recorded correctly, cases of lung cancer could in fact be classified as non-cases. Both of these situations introduce information bias. Both would bias the odds ratio towards 1 (null) because more 'noise' is introduced into the data.

Information bias can happen unintentionally and for many reasons, including:

- Data quality. Data entry errors, data coding errors, faulty equipment.

- Interviewer bias. Interviewers may be unintentionally more accurate for participants with diseases than for healthy participants, particularly common in case-control studies (Chapter 10).

- Recall bias. Participants asked to recall past events may not be accurate, particularly worrying in retrospective cohort studies that are concerned with exposures in the past.

- Reporting bias. Participants may over- or under-report exposures. For example, patients with brain tumours may be more likely to report greater mobile phone usage than those without. Pregnant women may under-report smoking given that smoking during pregnancy is not recommended and is stigmatised. Awareness/media bias can also encourage reporting bias.

Consider the following hypothetical data in Table A.1, in which two different methods for classifying smoking status were used, in an occupational cohort study. People were asked to report their own smoking status (self-report) and one of their colleagues was asked to report the participants' smoking status (informant-reported). Both kinds of report were compared to a gold standard (salivary cotinine). Using the generalised notation for diagnostic tests shown below, we can calculate the sensitivity and specificity of the self-report 'test' compared to the gold standard.

It was found that self-reported smoking status was reasonably accurate, having high sensitivity (most smokers, but not all, reported that they were smokers) and perfect specificity (no non-smokers said that they smoked). Ten smokers self-reported as non-smokers, reducing sensitivity. As you might

Table A.1 Notation for diagnostic tests

Generalised notation for diagnostic tests	Gold standard positive	Gold standard negative	Total
Test positive	a	b	e
Test negative	c	d	f
Total	g	h	N

Table A.2 Self-reported vs. informant-reported smoking

	Self-reported smoking compared to gold standard			Informant-reported smoking compared to gold standard		
	Smoker (salivary cotinine)	Non-smoker (salivary cotinine)	Total	Smoker (salivary cotinine)	Non-smoker (salivary cotinine)	Total
Self-reported smoker	90	0	90	80	0	80
Self-reported non-smoker	10	400	410	20	400	420
Total	100	400	500	100	400	500
	Sensitivity = 90% Specificity = 100% PPV = 92% NPV = 97%			Sensitivity = 80% Specificity = 100% PPV = 100% NPV = 95%		

expect, informant-reported smoking status was less accurate. Sensitivity was lower, because fewer smokers were identified as smokers by their colleagues. Smoking is increasingly discouraged, and can be a stigmatised behaviour. It can be hidden from colleagues, who may not be aware that this person smoked. Both methods lead to misclassification bias, although this is less problematic for self-report than for informant reports.

Misclassification of exposure status can bias the odds ratio towards no association. We can see this when calculating the odds ratio across the three scenarios: having salivary cotinine data (the gold standard, providing the true OR), having self-report data and having informant-report data. You can see that the greater the degree of misclassification bias, the more the association is pushed towards 1. The informant-report OR is only 1.86, much lower than the true OR of 4.75. This scenario assumes that the misclassification is the same across disease/healthy groups and that no other confounding is present. In reality, misclassification might be different among disease/healthy groups, further distorting the true effect.

Misclassification occurs when the sensitivity or the specificity of the measure used to ascertain exposure status becomes lower. As shown in the example above, the lower the sensitivity of a test, the more the association is pushed towards null. Similarly, the figure shows that the lower the specificity of a test, the more the association is pushed to null. When sensitivity and specificity are low (0.50 each), the apparent RR is 1. To summarise, left unchecked, information bias can distort the apparent association between risk factor x and outcome y. It is important to measure exposure status accurately, to reduce bias.

Table A.3 Gold standard, self-report and informant-report odds ratios

	Salivary cotinine			Self-report			Informant-report		
	Disease	Healthy	Total	Disease	Healthy	Total	Disease	Healthy	Total
Smoker	380	20	400	385	25	410	390	30	420
Non-smoker	80	20	100	75	15	90	70	10	80
Total	460	40	500	460	40	500	460	40	500
	$OR_{true} = ad/bc$			$OR = ad/bc$			$OR = ad/bc$		
	$OR_{true} = 4.75$			$OR = 3.08$			$OR = 1.86$		

Glossary

ADAS-cog A cognitive test battery designed to measure cognitive function, often used in RCTs. It is often considered more reliable and valid than MMSE.

Adjustment An association between an exposure and outcome can be adjusted for confounding factors, in order to reduce the distorting effect of the confounder on the association (see Chapter 6).

All-cause mortality Deaths from any cause.

Antagonism The combined effect of two exposures is smaller (e.g. less harmful) than the effect anticipated by one of them. The effect modifier 'cancels out' some of the risk. Biologic or real-world interaction means one of two things happens when the risk factors are combined: *antagonism* or *synergism*.

Cause-specific mortality Deaths from specific causes; for example, often grouped into the major causes of death (cardiovascular and cancer mortality).

Centring Subtracting the mean from x so that 0 represents the mean value of x (and the intercept represents the expected value of y when x is at its mean).

Charlson index A score reflecting the number and severity of co-morbidities. The original scale assigned a score of 1/2/3/6 for different conditions. The scale has since been revised, because survival probabilities have changed (e.g. AIDS mortality has decreased, cancer mortality has increased).

Cochrane Reviews Systematic reviews of primary research in human health care and health policy, and are internationally recognised as the highest standard in evidence-based health care. They investigate the effects of interventions for prevention, treatment and rehabilitation. They also assess the accuracy of a diagnostic test for a given condition in a specific patient group and setting. They are published online in the Cochrane Library.

Cognitive behavioural therapy (CBT) A type of psychotherapy which aims to change cognitions and behaviours by using a systematic approach that replaces patterns of thinking and reacting with more adaptive responses.

Complex interventions Interventions with several interacting components, which may not be standardised in delivery, and may be sensitive to local contexts. Complex interventions may have lengthy causal chains between the intervention and outcome.

Consolidated Standards of Reporting Trials (CONSORT) Statement An evidence-based set of recommendations and reporting requirements for RCTs. The guidelines provide a standard way to report results, and should be followed in papers submitted for publication.

Cotinine A metabolite of nicotine, used as a biomarker of exposure to tobacco. Salivary cotinine is thought to better reflect actual exposure than self-reported cigarettes smoked per day, for example.

Cox Regression A type of regression model that deals with time to event data (e.g. survival time before death). The model has to 'censor' participants who have not experienced the event before the end of follow-up, because they might still experience the event. Typical outcomes for Cox Regression models include all-cause mortality, cause-specific mortality, cancer and infection.

Cumulative exposure Exposures which happen more often, for longer periods, and are more severe, may result in cumulative damage to biological systems or psychological outcomes. Accordingly, it can be useful to collect information about exposures over many years (e.g. pack years of smoking).

Dose-response association When an increase in the exposure strengthens the size of the association between the exposure and outcome, and a decrease weakens it. For example, smoking has a dose-response association with lung cancer because smoking more cigarettes increases risk in lung cancer.

Effectiveness The benefit of an intervention under normal 'real world' conditions, in practice or routine situations.

Efficacy The benefit of an intervention under 'ideal' conditions, such as RCTs. Efficacy is not the same as effectiveness (see effectiveness).

Efficiency The impact on outcomes in terms of the resources used. When efficacy and effectiveness are known, efficiency is a measure of the cost of achieving this impact.

Freedom of information Any person requesting information from a public authority is entitled (a) to be informed about whether or not this information exists and is held; (b) if it is held, to have the information communicated to them.

Google Scholar A free web search engine, covering the scholarly literature.

Grey literature Literature that has not been through the formal peer-review and commercial publication process. For example, reports, grant applications, technical papers, working papers.

Hawthorne effect When awareness of being in a study changes the outcome, usually improving it. This can apply to treatment or control groups, and is not addressed by randomisation. Effects can be over-estimated in treatment and control groups because there is some benefit to participating in the research, whatever the reason.

Health selection When participants are selected, typically at recruitment, on characteristics that produce a healthier sample than the wider population.

Healthy survivor effects A form of selection attrition whereby healthier participants tend to remain in the study. Smokers for example, will tend to die and drop-out from a study, producing a sample that contains healthier smokers than in the population (a 'healthy' smoker effect) [4].

Hierarchy of evidence Study designs are ranked according to the quality or reliability of the evidence they can provide: RCT, cohort, case-control, observational or cross-sectional

Incidence rate ratio This is a relative measure of the greater/smaller incidence in rate in an exposed group, compared to an unexposed group. For example, if the rate of a new infection is 0.002 in an exposed group, 0.001 in an unexposed group, then the incidence rate ratio is 2. The rate of infection is twice as high.

Index Medicus Prior to 1979, the National Library of Medicine (NLM) used a printed record called *Index Medicus*.

Interaction Statistical interaction means that the combined association is greater than the sum of the two separate exposures. This can be protective or harmful.

Intentional to treat (ITT) analysis A method of analysing results from randomised controlled trials where participants are analysed according to the original treatment intention. Some participants may be lost to follow-up or change treatment groups, as often happens in real clinical practice, and so an ITT analysis takes this into consideration.

Intercept The predicted/estimated value of y when $x=0$. The 'origin' of the line of best fit.

International Classification of Diseases (ICD) A diagnostic tool which applies standard codes to diseases and other health problems, including mortality records.

Lung age The age of the average person with a forced expiratory volume in one second (FEV_1) value the same as the individual. Considered a 'biomarker' of lung function.

MEDLINE The National Library of Medicine in the USA has been indexing medical literature since 1979.

Mini Mental State Examination (MMSE) MMSE scores range from 0 (worst possible score) to 30 (best possible score) and 25+ is considered normal. Various cut points for categorising people have been proposed, and are debated, but for illustrative purposes: 25 or more = normal, 18 to 24 = mild to moderate cognitive impairment, 17 or less = serious impairment. Age and educational attainment may influence MMSE score, which should be kept in mind.

Misclassification When a value is put into the wrong category. For example, if a non-smoker is classified as a smoker, they have been misclassified.

Multiple imputation A method for addressing missing data by estimating the missing values and replacing them, often resulting in multiple datasets which are each analysed and the results combined.

Multiple risk When two risk factors increase risk, either because of their additive effects (e.g. if 2 + 2 = 4) or because of a synergistic *interaction* (e.g. if 2 + 2 = 6).

Narrative review These are often used in expert summaries, student dissertations, polemics, talks and opinion articles[2]. Studies are selected by the author with no explicit search or inclusion criteria.

Negative predictive value (NPV) Proportion of people with a negative result who actually are negative (d/f).

Number needed to harm (NNH). Number of patients needed to be treated for one additional patient to be harmed (NNH). A measure of clinical significance. 1/(1–OR)UER (UER = unexposed event rate). Number needed to treat (NNT) is the equivalent in reverse.

Poisson distribution A distribution seen with count data, having a peak and a long tail. Shows how many discrete events have occurred in a given time period.

Positive predictive value (PPV) Proportion of people with a positive result who actually are positive (a/e).

Public Health Observatories Public Health Observatories (PHOs) produce information, data and intelligence on people's health and health care for practitioners, commissioners, policy makers and the wider community (see www.apho.org.uk).

Public interest test If releasing information is in the public interest, it is considered to service the interests of the public. An example of when releasing information would not be in the public interest, would be to release information that would prevent prosecution of an offender. Crucially, the public interest test does not refer to things which are interesting to the public.

Recall bias When a self-report, usually relating to an exposure, is inaccurate or incomplete. This introduces systematic error into the measure.

Regression line Line added, usually to a scatter plot, showing the expected value of an outcome variable according to the predictor variable, and a line of best fit that best illustrates the relationship between the two variables.

Regression to the mean The tendency of values at the tails of a distribution to move closer to the mean at the next measurement occasion.

Research ethics The moral principles guiding research from its inception through to completion and publication of results [1].

Reverse causation When the supposed exposure is actually influenced by the supposed outcome, rather than vice versa.

Sensitivity The proportion of people with the result correctly identified by the measure (a/g).

Slope. The predicted/estimated change in y when x increases by 1 unit. The 'gradient' of the line of best fit.

Specificity The proportion of people without the result correctly identified by the measure (d/h).

Standardised regression coefficient Predicted standard deviation change in y per standard deviation increase in x.

Surrogate endpoint Surrogate endpoints or markers of variables (e.g. blood pressure) which might correlate highly with the real clinical endpoint (e.g. heart disease) and are used as a substitution.

Synergism The combined risk is stronger (e.g. more harmful) than the sum of the two separate risks. The effect modifier strengthens some of the risk. This is equivalent to 'effect modification' when one exposure modifies the risk of another (Chapter 6). It may not be immediately obvious which variable is the supposed causal variable and which is the modifier. They may modify each others' risks.

Threshold effect When there is an association between an exposure and an outcome above a certain threshold value, but no association below this threshold.

Time-varying confounding Time-varying variables which are confounding factors, may introduce time-varying confounding. Allowing interactions between a confounding factor and time can be used to adjust for time-varying confounders. Obviously, this means that the variables need to have been measured repeatedly over time, which is often not done in cohort studies.

Ulrich's Periodicals Directory A database of popular and academic journals, magazines, newspapers and periodicals. http://www.serialssolutions.com/en/services/ulrichs

References

1. British Psychological Society: *Code of Human Research Ethics*. Leicester: BPS; 2010.
2. Torgerson C: *Systematic Reviews*. London: Continuum International Publishing Group; 2003.
3. Gerstman BB: *Basic Biostatics: Statistics for Public Health Practice*. Sudbury, MA: Jones and Bartlett Publishers, Inc; 2008.
4. Becklake MR, Lalloo U: The 'healthy smoker': a phenomenon of health selection? *Respiration: International Review of Thoracic Diseases* 1990, 57(3):137–144.
5. Bignold S: *A review of linking teaching and research in the health sciences and practice disciplines*. London: LTSN Centre for Health Sciences and Practice 2003.
6. Long A, Harrison S: Evidence-based decision making. *Health Service Journal* 1997, S6:1–11.
7. Evidence-based Medicine Working Group: Evidence-based medicine. A new approach to teaching the practice of medicine. *JAMA: The Journal of the American Medical Association* 1992, 268(17):2420–2425.
8. Porzsolt F, Ohletz A, Thim A, Gardner D, Ruatti H, Meier H, Schlotz-Gorton N, Schrott L: Evidence-based decision making: the six step approach. *Evidence Based Medicine* 2003, 8(6):165–166.
9. Nicol DJ, Macfarlane-Dick D: Formative assessment and self-regulated learning: a model and seven principles of good feedback practice. *Studies in Higher Education* 2006, 31(2):199 - 218.
10. Lipkus I, Samsa G, Rimer B: General performance on a numeracy scale among highly educated samples. *Medical Decision Making* 2001, 21(1):37–44.
11. Schwartz LM, Woloshin S, Black WC, Welch HG: The role of numeracy in understanding the benefit of screening mammography. *Annals Internal Medicine* 1997, 127(11):966–972.
12. Allerhand M: *A Tiny Handbook of R* (SpringerBriefs in Statistics). Heidelberg: Springer: ; 2011.
13. Bittinger M: *Basic College Mathematics*. London: Pearson Education; 2009.
14. Johnson T, Neill H: *Teach Yourself Mathematics*, 3rd edn. London: Teach Yourself; 2008.
15. Crawley M: *The R Book*. Chichester: Wiley; 2012.
16. Field A, Miles J, Field Z: *Discovering Statistics Using R*: Thousand Oaks, CA: SAGE Publications Ltd; 2012.
17. Graham A: *Teach Yourself Statistics*. London:Teach Yourself; 2003.
18. Velleman P, Wilkinson L: Nominal, ordinal, interval, and ratio typologies are misleading. *The American Statistician* 1993, 47(1):65–72.
19. Miles J, Shevlin M: *Applying Regression and Correlation: A Guide for Students and Researchers*. Thousand Oaks, CA: SAGE Publications Ltd; 2000.
20. Kirkwood BR, Sterne JAC: *Essential Medical Statistics*, 2nd edn. Oxford: Blackwell; 2003.
21. Craig R, Mindell J, Hirani V: *Health Survey for England – 2008 trend tables*. London: UCL; 2008.

22. Bartlett AA: Logarithmic scales: a useful example. *The Physics Teacher* 2003, 41:16–17.

23. Sedgwick P, Hall A: Teaching medical students and doctors how to communicate risk. *British Medical Journal* 2003, 327(7417):694–695.

24. Cornfield J, Haenszel W, Hammond C, Lilienfeld A, Shimkin M, Wynder E: Smoking and lung cancer: recent evidence and a discussion of some questions. *International Journal of Epidemiology* 2009, 38(5):1175–1191.

25. Akobeng AK: Understanding measures of treatment effect in clinical trials. *Archives of Diseases in Childhood* 2005, 90(1):54–56.

26. Edwards PJRI, Clarke MJ, DiGuiseppi C, Wentz R, Kwan I, Cooper R, Felix LM, Pratap S. : Methods to increase response to postal and electronic questionnaires. *Cochrane Database of Systematic Reviews* 2009, 3:MR000008.

27. Islami F, Pourshams A, Nasrollahzadeh D, Kamangar F, Fahimi S, Shakeri R, Abedi-Ardekani B, Merat S, Vahedi H, Semnani S *et al:* Tea drinking habits and oesophageal cancer in a high risk area in northern Iran: population based case-control study. *British Medical Journal* 2009, 338: b929.

28. Kemmeren J, Algra A, Grobbee D: Third generation oral contraceptives and risk of venous thrombosis: meta-analysis. *British Medical Journal* 2001, 323:131.

29. Shickle D: "On a supposed right to lie [to the public] from benevolent motives": communicating health risks to the public. *Medicine, Health Care, and Philosophy* 2000, 3(3):241–249.

30. Scott I, Mazhindu D: *Statistics for Health Care Professionals.* London: SAGE; 2005.

31. Sholer F: *Type I, II and III Sums of Squares* [http://goanna.cs.rmit.edu.au/~fscholer/anova.php]

32. Salkind N: *Statistics for People Who (Think They) Hate Statistics.* Los Angeles, CA: Sage Publications, Inc; 2010.

33. Hagger-Johnson G, Bewick B, Conner M, O'Connor D, Shickle D: Alcohol, conscientiousness and event-level condom use. *British Journal of Health Psychology* 2011, 16(4):828–845.

34. Singh-Manoux A: Commentary: modelling multiple pathways to explain social inequalities in health and mortality. *International Journal of Epidemiology* 2005, 34(3):638–639.

35. Holst PA, Kromhout D, Brand R: For debate: pet birds as an independent risk factor for lung cancer. *British Medical Journal* 1988, 297(6659):1319–1321.

36. Britton J, Lewis S: Pet birds and lung cancer. *British Medical Journal* 1996, 313(7067):1218–1219.

37. Gardiner A, Lee P: Pet birds and lung cancer. *British Medical Journal (Clinical Research Ed)* 1993, 306(6869).

38. Modigh C, Axelsson G, Alavanja M, Andersson L, Rylander R: Pet birds and risk of lung cancer in Sweden: a case-control study. *British Medical Journal* 1996, 313(7067):1236–1238.

39. Kohlmeier L, Arminger G, Bartolomeycik S, Bellach B, Rehm J, Thamm M: Pet birds as an independent risk factor for lung cancer: case-control study. *British Medical Journal (Clinical Research Ed)* 1992, 305(6860):986–989.

40. Li Y-F: *Confounding, Effect Modification and Stratification* (presentation) [http://www.docstoc.com/docs/145754038/Confounding_-Effect-Modification_-and-Stratification]

41. World Health Organization: *Reducing risks, promoting healthy life.* Geneva: World Health Organization; 2002.

42. Baron R, Kenny D: The moderator-mediator variable distinction in social psychological research: conceptual, strategic, and statistical considerations. *Journal of Personality and Social Psychology* 1986, 51(6):1173–1182.

43. Bradford Hill A: The environment and disease: association or causation? *Proceedings of the Royal Society of Medicine* 1965, 58:295–300.

44. Doll R, Peto R, Boreham J, Sutherland I: Mortality in relation to smoking: 50 years' observations on male British doctors. *British Medical Journal* 2004, 328(7455):1519.

45. Cancer Research UK: *Lung cancer mortality statistics* [http://www.cancerresearchuk. org/cancer-info/cancerstats/types/lung/mortality/uk-lung-cancer-mortality-statistics]

46. Khuder SA: Effect of cigarette smoking on major histological types of lung cancer: a meta-analysis. *Lung Cancer* 2001, 31(2–3):139–148.

47. Rothman K: Causes. *American Journal of Epidemiology* 1976, 104:587–592.

48. Rothman K, Greenland S: *Modern Epidemiology*, 2nd edn. Philadelphia, PA: Lippincott-Raven; 1998.

49. Hagger-Johnson G, McManus J, Hutchison C, Barker M: Building partnerships with the voluntary sector. *Psychologist* 2003, 19:156–158.

50. McDonald S, Taylor L, Adams C: Searching the right database. A comparison of four databases for psychiatry journals. *Health Libraries Review* 1999, 16(3):151–156.

51. Altman DG, Schulz KF, Moher D, Egger M, Davidoff F, Elbourne D, Gotzsche PC, Lang T, Grp C: The revised CONSORT statement for reporting randomized trials: explanation and elaboration. *Annals of Internal Medicine* 2001, 134(8):663–694.

52. Imrie J, Stephenson JM, Cowan FM, Wanigaratne S, Billington AJ, Copas AJ, French L, French PD, Johnson AM, Behavioural Intervention in Gay Men Project Study G: A cognitive behavioural intervention to reduce sexually transmitted infections among gay men: randomised trial. *British Medical Journal* 2001, 322(7300):1451–1456.

53. Glick SN, Morris M, Foxman B, Aral SO, Manhart LE, Holmes KK, Golden MR: A comparison of sexual behavior patterns among men who have sex with men and heterosexual men and women. *Journal of Acquired Immune Deficiency Syndromes* 2012, 60(1):83–90.

54. Hart GJ, Williamson LM, Flowers P: Good in parts: the Gay Men's Task Force in Glasgow - a response to Kelly. *AIDS Care – Psychological Socio-Medical Aspects of AIDS/HIV* 2004, 16(2):159–165.

55. Anderson R: New MRC guidance on evaluating complex interventions. *British Medical Journal* 2008, 337.

56. Richens J, Imrie J, Copas A: Condoms and seat belts: the parallels and the lessons. *Lancet* 2000, 355(9201):400–403.

57. Parkes G, Greenhalgh T, Griffin M, Dent R: Effect on smoking quit rate of telling patients their lung age: the Step2quit randomised controlled trial. *British Medical Journal* 2008, 336(7644):598–600.

58. McClure JB: Are biomarkers a useful aid in smoking cessation? A review and analysis of the literature. *Behavioral Medicine* 2001, 27(1):37–47.

59. Lautenschlager Nt CKLFL, et al.: Effect of physical activity on cognitive function in older adults at risk for alzheimer disease: A randomized trial. *JAMA: The Journal of the American Medical Association* 2008, 300(9):1027–1037.

60. World Health Organization: *Global Recommendations on Physical Activity for Health: 65 Years and Above*. Geneva: WHO; 2011.

61. Buchman AS, Boyle PA, Yu L, Shah RC, Wilson RS, Bennett DA: Total daily physical activity and the risk of AD and cognitive decline in older adults. *Neurology* 2012, 78(17):1323–1329.

62. Singh-Manoux A, Kivimaki M, Glymour MM, Elbaz A, Berr C, Ebmeier KP, Ferrie JE, Dugravot A: Timing of onset of cognitive decline: results from Whitehall II prospective cohort study. *British Medical Journal* 2012, 344.

63. Reid L, MacLullich A: Subjective memory complaints and cognitive impairment in older people. *Dementia and Geriatric Cognitive Disorders* 2006, 22(5–6):471–485.

64. Enstrom J, Kabat G: Environmental tobacco smoke and tobacco related mortality in a prospective study of Californians, 1960–98. *British Medical Journal* 2003, 326(7398):1057.

65. Enstrom JE, Heath CW: Smoking cessation and mortality trends among 118,000 Californians, 1960–1997. *Epidemiology (Cambridge, MA)* 1999, 10(5):500–512.

66. Garfinkel L: Selection, follow-up, and analysis in the American Cancer Society prospective studies. *National Cancer Institute monograph* 1985, 67:49–52.

67. Shor E, Roelfs D, Curreli M, Clemow L, Burg M, Schwartz J: Widowhood and mortality: a meta-analysis and meta-regression. *Demography* 2012, 49(2):575–606.

68. Taylor R, Najafi F, Dobson A: Meta-analysis of studies of passive smoking and lung cancer: effects of study type and continent. *International Journal of Epidemiology* 2007, 36(5):1048–1059.

69. Xu W-H, Zhang X-L, Gao Y-T, Xiang Y-B, Gao L-F, Zheng W, Shu X-O: Joint effect of cigarette smoking and alcohol consumption on mortality. *Preventive medicine* 2007, 45(4):313–319.

70. Altman DG, Bland JM: Interaction revisited: the difference between two estimates. *British Medical Journal* 2003, 326(7382):219.

71. Altman DG, Matthews JNS: Statistics Notes: Interaction 1: Heterogeneity of effects. *British Medical Journal* 1996, 313(7055):486.

72. Matthews JNS, Altman DG: Statistics Notes: Interaction 2: Compare effect sizes not P values. *British Medical Journal* 1996, 313(7060):808.

73. Matthews JNS, Altman DG: Statistics notes: Interaction 3: How to examine heterogeneity. *British Medical Journal* 1996, 313(7061):862.

74. Rothman K, Greenland S, Walker A: Concepts of interaction. *American Journal of Epidemiology* 1980, 112(4):467–470.

75. Taylor B, Rehm J: When risk factors combine: the interaction between alcohol and smoking for aerodigestive cancer, coronary heart disease, and traffic and fire injury. *Addictive behaviors* 2006, 31(9):1522–1535.

76. Zeka A, Gore R, Kriebel D: Effects of alcohol and tobacco on aerodigestive cancer risks: a meta-regression analysis. *Cancer Causes & Control: CCC* 2003, 14(9):897–906.

77. Gmel G, Daeppen JB: Recall bias for seven-day recall measurement of alcohol consumption among emergency department patients: Implications for case-crossover designs. *Journal of Studies on Alcohol and Drugs* 2007, 68(2):303–310.

78. Shaper AG, Wannamethee G, Walker M: Alcohol and mortality in British men - explaining the U-shaped curve. *Lancet* 1988, 2(8623):1267–1273.

79. Reidy J, McHugh E, Stassen LFA: A review of the relationship between alcohol and oral cancer. *Surgeon: Journal of the Royal College of Surgeons of Edinburgh and Ireland* 2011, 9(5):278–283.

80. Gronbaek M, Becker U, Johansen D, Gottschau A, Schnohr P, Hein HO, Jensen G, Sorensen TIA: Type of alcohol consumed and mortality from all causes, coronary heart disease, and cancer. *Annals of Internal Medicine* 2000, 133(6):411–419.

81. Ronksley P, Brien S, Turner B, Mukamal K, Ghali W: Association of alcohol consumption with selected cardiovascular disease outcomes: a systematic review and meta-analysis. *British Medical Journal* 2011, 342.

82. Hart C, Davey Smith G, Gruer L, Watt G: The combined effect of smoking tobacco and drinking alcohol on cause-specific mortality: a 30 year cohort study. *BMC Public Health* 2010, 10(1):789.

83. Lin H, Ng S, Chan S, Chan W, Lee K, Ho S, Tian L: Institutional risk factors for norovirus outbreaks in Hong Kong elderly homes: a retrospective cohort study. *BMC Public Health* 2011, 11(1):297.

84. Babyak M: What you see may not be what you get: a brief, nontechnical introduction to overfitting in regression-type models. *Psychosomatic Medicine* 2004, 66(3):411–421.

85. Boffetta P: Internal and external validity of cohort studies. *Annals of Agricultural and Environmental Medicine: AAEM* 2011, 18(2):283–284.

86. Bernaards CM, Twisk JW, Snel J, Van Mechelen W, Kemper HC: Is calculating pack-years retrospectively a valid method to estimate life-time tobacco smoking? A comparison between prospectively calculated pack-years and retrospectively calculated pack-years. *Addiction (Abingdon, UK)* 2001, 96(11):1653–1661.

87. Alavanja MC, Brownson RC, Berger E, Lubin J, Modigh C: Avian exposure and risk of lung cancer in women in Missouri: population based case-control study. *British Medical Journal* 1996, 313(7067):1233–1235.

88. Stacey T, Thompson JMD, Mitchell EA, Ekeroma AJ, Zuccollo JM, McCowan LME: Association between maternal sleep practices and risk of late stillbirth: a case-control study. *British Medical Journal* 2011, 342:d3403.

89. Bjerre LM, LeLorier J: Expressing the magnitude of adverse effects in case-control studies: "The number of patients needed to be treated for one additional patient to be harmed". *British Medical Journal (Clinical Research Ed)* 2000, 320(7233):503–506.

90. Aydin D, Feychting M, Schüz J, Tynes T, Andersen TV, Schmidt LS, Poulsen AH, Johansen C, Prochazka M, Lannering B *et al:* Mobile phone use and brain tumors in children and adolescents: a multicenter case–control study. *Journal of the National Cancer Institute* 2011, 103(16):1264–1276.

91. Boice JD, Tarone RE: Cell phones, cancer, and children. *Journal of the National Cancer Institute* 2011, 103(16):1211–1213.

92. Ahlbom A, Feychting M, Green A, Kheifets L, Savitz D, Swerdlow A: Epidemiologic evidence on mobile phones and tumor risk: a review. *Epidemiology (Cambridge, MA)* 2009, 20(5):639–652.

93. Christ A, Gosselin M-C, Christopoulou M, Kühn S, Kuster N: Age-dependent tissue-specific exposure of cell phone users. *Physics in Medicine and Biology* 2010, 55(7):1767.

94. Wiart J, Hadjem A, Wong MF, Bloch I: Analysis of RF exposure in the head tissues of children and adults. *Physics in Medicine and Biology* 2008, 53(13):3681–3695.

95. Medical Research Council: *Good research practice: principles and guidelines.* Swindon: Medical Research Council; 2012.

96. Miles J: A framework for power analysis using a structural equation modelling procedure. *BMC Medical Research Methodology* 2003, 3(1):27.

97. Boynton PM: Administering, analysing, and reporting your questionnaire. *British Medical Journal* 2004, 328(7452):1372–1375.

98. Boynton PM, Greenhalgh T: Selecting, designing, and developing your questionnaire. *British Medical Journal* 2004, 328(7451):1312–1315.

99. Boynton PM, Wood GW, Greenhalgh T, Clinic Q: Reaching beyond the white middle classes. *British Medical Journal* 2004, 328(7453):1433–1436.

100. Information Commissioner: The public interest test: Freedom of Information Act. London: Information Commisioner's Office; 2013 [http://ico.org.uk/for_organisations/guidance_index/~/media/documents/library/Freedom_of_Information/Detailed_specialist_guides/the_public_interest_test.ashx].

101. Marmot M, Brunner E: Cohort profile: The Whitehall II cohort study. *International Journal of Epidemiology* 2005, 34(2):251–256.

102. Sabia S, Elbaz A, Dugravot A, Head J, Shipley M, Hagger-Johnson G, Kivimaki M, Singh-Manoux A: Impact of smoking on cognitive decline in early old age: The Whitehall II cohort study. *Archives of General Psychiatry* 2012: 69(6):627–635..

103. Katzmarzyk P, Church T, Craig C, Bouchard C: Sitting time and mortality from all causes, cardiovascular disease, and cancer. *Medicine and Science in Sports and Exercise* 2009, 41(5):998–1005.

104. Prina AM, Huisman M, Yeap BB, Hankey GJ, Flicker L, Brayne C, Almeida OP: Association between depression and hospital outcomes among older men. *Canadian Medical Association Journal* 2012: 185(2):117–123.

105. Tabachnick B, Fidell L: *Using Multivariate Statistics*: Boston, MA: Bacon & Allyn; 2007.

106. Daabiss M: American Society of Anaesthesiologists physical status classification. *Indian Journal of Anaesthesia* 2011, 55(2):111–115.

107. Hosmer D, Lemeshow S: *Applied Logistic Regression*: Chichester: Wiley Interscience; 2000.

108. Jüni P, Altman D, Egger M: Assessing the quality of controlled clinical trials. *British Medical Journal* 2001, 323(7303):42–46.

109. Carlson M, Morrison S: Study design, precision, and validity in observational studies. *Journal of Palliative Medicine* 2009, 12(1):77–82.

110. Bayona M, Olsen C.: *Observational Studies and Bias in Epidemiology* [http://www.collegeboard.com/prod_downloads/yes/4297_MODULE_19.pdf]

111. Feinstein AR, Walter SD, Horwitz RI: An analysis of Berkson's bias in case-control studies. *Journal of Chronic Diseases* 1986, 39(7):495–504.

112. Moffatt S, Mulloli TP, Bhopal R, Foy C, Phillimore P: An exploration of awareness bias in two environmental epidemiology studies. *Epidemiology (Cambridge, MA)* 2000, 11(2):199–208.

113. Szklo M, Nieto J: *Epidemiology: Beyond the Basics*: Sudbury, MA: Jones and Bartlett Publishers; 2006.

114. Copeland K, Checkoway H, McMichael A, Holbrook R: Bias due to misclassification in the estimation of relative risk. *American Journal of Epidemiology* 1977, 105(5):488–495.

115. Langdridge D, Hagger-Johnson G: *Introduction to Research Methods and Data Analysis in Psychology*: 2nd edn, Harlow: Prentice Hall; 2009

116. Critical Appraisal Skills Programme: Making sense of evidence [http://www.casp-uk.net/]

Index

Italic page numbers indicate tables; bold indicate figures.

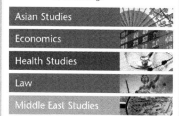